MALPRACTICE IN MADISON

BREAKING THE CODE OF SILENCE
A WHISTLEBLOWER'S STORY
EXPOSES SELECTIVE STUPIDITY

Dr. Ira Williams

Author's Tranquility Press
ATLANTA, GEORGIA

Copyright © 2023 by Dr. Ira Williams

All rights reserved. No part of this publication may be reproduced, distributed or transmitted in any form or by any means, including photocopying, recording, or other electronic or mechanical methods, without the prior written permission of the publisher, except in the case of brief quotations embodied in critical reviews and certain other noncommercial uses permitted by copyright law. For permission requests, write to the publisher, addressed "Attention: Permissions Coordinator," at the address below.

Dr. Ira Williams/Author's Tranquility Press
3800 Camp Creek Pkwy SW Bldg. 1400-116 #1255
Atlanta, GA 30331, USA
www.authorstranquilitypress.com

Publisher's Note: This is a work of documented non-fiction. The views and insights presented in this book represent the author's expertise and research, and they are intended to stimulate meaningful discussions and expand our understanding of the subject matter. The content within these pages has been carefully curated to provide readers with a comprehensive exploration that contributes to the ongoing dialogue on important topics.

Ordering Information:
Quantity sales. Special discounts are available on quantity purchases by corporations, associations, and others. For details, contact the "Special Sales Department" at the address above.

Malpractice In Madison/Dr. Ira Williams
Paperback: 978-1-961908-95-6
eBook: 978-1-961908-96-3

Contents

Foreword i
Introduction viii
Agnes 1
Drs. Tom and Tim 7
Medical Peer Review 15
Medical Peer Review Ends 37
Healthcare Stupidity 63
Foreword 68
Foreword—Donald M. Berwick, MD
Institute for Healthcare Improvement 70
Preface 71
Medical Malpractice 97
Organized Medicine 115
State Medical Examining Boards 117
A Brief History of Health Care 122
A 21st Century HCDS 146
Real Healthcare 149
Three Greatest Healthcare Mistakes 151
2020 Preface 155

Foreword

This is my fifth book on the Healthcare Delivery System (doctors & hospitals), and I am the only Quality of Care and Patient Safety expert saying the following:

> **I know Why the current HCDS is and has always been broken.**
>
> **I know How the current HCDS is and has always been broken.**
>
> More importantly
>
> **I know How to begin to create a 21st century HCDS, and no one seems interested.**

How could a dentist, board certified oral & maxillofacial surgeon and anesthesiologist, but still, just a dentist, become an expert on Your & Your Loved One's Healthcare Delivery System (HCDS)? Well, it wasn't easy, and I paid a huge price, but I made the right life-changing decision, and I have never looked back with regret, and perhaps the step-by-step process, and year-by year series of events that have enabled me to make the above collection of claims might prove interesting to some. My evolution into becoming a HCDS expert was not planned, but the process has served to define me.

Agnes, a middle-aged, wife and mother living in Baraboo Wisconsin would, unintentionally, set in motion the series of events that would lead to my becoming the anthesis to the desired characteristics of a member of the medical and dental professions, and a positive contrarian challenging the long-standing efforts to improve the Quality of Care and Patient Safety within mine and your current, and highly flawed, Healthcare Delivery System.

Leadership within the Medical and Dental Professions, at local, state, and national levels have always demanded that each practitioner adhere to the Code of Silence regarding issues of questionable patient care provided by a fellow member of their profession. This well-established Code of Silence can be suspended in rare instances, particularly at the local level of the professions, and I was the beneficiary of one such incidence in Madison, and an active participant in another such incidence, but while both professions will celebrate such events, those same sources will choose to ignore their rarity. That brief contrast of professional, or more accurately, unprofessional behavior leads to a basic understanding.

The overwhelming reliance on the Code of Silence is the basic reason Why and How the current Healthcare Delivery System is and has always been broken! How?

Medical Leadership has always been lying to the Public, and the Code of Silence has always been the foundation for those lies throughout the history of that Profession, and the evidence for such a claim is plentiful, and clearly evident to those who desire such an understanding, as I have done for over 40 years, by reading and studying that history.

Pasteur opened the door to Modern Medicine in the late 19th century, and a study of his activities in the process of his opening that door is dominated by the medical leadership of his day in their efforts to obstruct and vilify his efforts, until his successes forced them to suddenly accept his expertise, and begin to save more lives than they had been killing throughout the history of their Profession. Medical Leadership, even today, does not take kindly to those who wish to talk about the Dark Side of Medicine that continues today. But it is impossible to begin to understand current problems in that System while ignoring the Dark Side of the Professions.

I am in essence a classic whistleblower, and as such, I am not well received by my chosen profession, dentistry, or that other profession that has always dominated the healthcare systems throughout the world. And I have a well-established track record that supports my whistleblower claim.

Dr. Jeffrey Wigand achieved national prominence in 1995 when he became the tobacco industry's highest ranking former executive to finally begin to tell the truth about the health effects of smoking, and what the top leaders of that industry had always known. I am trying to do the same regarding the long-standing failures in how to begin to make the delivery of healthcare far safer.

Agnes was not only my first experience as one who would challenge the way hospital medical staff conduct their business, particularly when it comes to the unpleasant task of reviewing questionable patient care provided by one of their staff members. But more importantly, all the events of her story led me to recognize the need for someone to do just that, challenge the hospital medical system from within that system. And challenge it I did.

Agnes was the first of three separate patient-care occasions when I was caused to become the second surgeon tasked with the need to surgically correct a previous surgeon's highly negligent care, and simultaneously breaking the Code of Silence within the community I practiced. Kamikaze pilots only flew one mission; I was tasked with three no-win situations within a few short years, and those in Madison who embraced the Code of Silence made sure that I paid the price for my insurrection.

But those experiences, and the unprofessional responses to what should have been judged to be my ethical and professional conduct caused me to make the decision that has allowed me to fully understand Why and How our current HCDS has always been far less than desired, and ultimately, able to write my books. One year after I was forced out of my group surgical practice, and found that I was now the only board-certified oral surgeon in Madison that was not allowed to become a member of the multiple HMOs that dominated the economics of patient care in that city I began to recognize that the price I would pay for my breaking the Code of Silence would be economic strangulation, and within a very few years the Medical and Dental Leadership in Madison gained their revenge. I was forced to leave Wisconsin, but not before I had set in motion the path for my future.

The first decision that redirected my life was when I agreed to become the only expert witness for Agnes and her husband in their medical malpractice suit.

The second, and possibly even greater decision was when I decided to advertise that I was available to act as a plaintiff's expert witness in oral surgery malpractice cases nationwide.

Now, not only did the medical and dental professionals in Madison hate me, but I had instantly become an enemy within my dental specialty. Not how to win friends and influence people.

I immediately received my first request to review a case of possible surgical negligence, and that case demonstrated all of the elements of how the Medical and Dental Leadership have completely corrupted every aspect of any attempt in judging questionable patient care by leaving the public with Sue or Forget It, while simultaneously demanding practitioners to adhere to the Code of Silence, and by *all of the elements,* I do mean all of the elements.

A well-established oral surgeon who was on the staff of the Ohio State University Oral Surgery Department attempted to surgically correct the jaw deformity for a middle-aged woman, and clearly demonstrated that he was unqualified to attempt surgery of that type. I reviewed the documents, photos, and x-rays of that case that had been sent to me by the patient's attorney, and I notified him that I was qualified to judge that patient's treatment as being negligent, and that I thought the facts of that case were so overwhelmingly negligent that I would be surprised if the surgeon and his malpractice insurer didn't agree and just settle the case. Boy, was I wrong, because all the predictable elements of medical malpractice litigation would rapidly come into play.

Chairman of Oral Surgery at the Wisconsin College of Medicine in Milwaukee would give a deposition and lie under oath that in his view the surgeon had done nothing wrong. The MD/DDS surgeon who had agreed to provide the patient with corrective surgery said he would do so, but he would not testify (break the Code of Silence) on her behalf. Her attorney concluded that he did not think I had sufficient standing necessary to overcome the false statement by that Chairman of Oral Surgery, and therefore also necessary to provide the burden of proof. Thus, the patient never got her day in court, and another example of surgical negligence fell into the win column for the Professions.

Yes, that case took place almost 40 years ago, and I have news for those who might think that that is too long ago. Nothing has changed regarding medical malpractice litigation except that all aspects of the critical elements of all patient care are even worse now, and no one seems to care.

I would go on to serve as a Plaintiff's expert witness in surgical malpractice cases in several states, including testifying as the Plaintiff's expert witness in downtown Boston, and against the Dean of Harvard Dental School. He and his residents in oral surgery had operated a middle-aged man for the surgical correction of a jaw deformity, and they had caused negligent harm during, and immediately after that surgery. But he had been elevated to become the new Dean of that dental school prior to the case being heard in court. The outcome was predictable; other experts testified that the harm to the patient was not negligence, and no judge in Boston was going to allow the Dean of Harvard Dental School to be found guilty of malpractice. The facts are the patient was harmed by that surgery, and the Profession got another win.

My experiences acting as a Plaintiff's expert witness in surgical malpractice litigation would prove to be extremely important in my efforts to better understand our current HCDS, and why and how it has fundamental deficiencies, but I will end this aspect of my journey seeking greater understanding with the latest, and very late experience as an expert witness.

2014 Ali, a young Muslim who was a recent graduate from law school in Southern California was told by someone who knew my background in such matters that he should call me. Ali had had surgical correction of a slight jaw deformity by an oral surgeon in Orange County CA, and that surgery had not gone well, and would I review his case documents for he and his attorney, and I said yes.

A brief recount of Ali's ordeal will hopefully be sufficient; his surgeon claimed to be dual degreed MD/DDS, but he had obtained his "MD" from a Caribbean medical school, and his degree was not recognized by any state. His surgeon had also turned what should have been a minor surgical correction into unnecessary double-jaw surgery, and with resultant major, harmful complications that resulted in a second surgery that was even more negligent. After three years of legal proceedings Ali and his attorney became faced with a major need. The surgeon's attorney and insurer claimed that there was no evidence of negligent care, and they sought dismissal of the case. The judge requested Ali and his attorney to offer proof of negligence, and Ali called me. I proceeded to document step-by-step every element of negligence in a seven-legal-page Declaration of Facts. The surgeon and his insurer immediately settled the case for the full amount, and I, at age 85 finally got a win for the good guys.

Whistleblowers must be created by actively participating inside that aspect of life that will enable them to forcibly challenge fundamental mismanagement, and while it has taken me several decades to become sufficiently qualified, I feel it is time for me to do so.

People need to wake up! Quality of Care and Patient Safety experts have been providing evidence of major flaws in Your & Your Loved One's Healthcare Delivery System for decades, and no one seems to care. Hopefully, one example will serve to illustrate such consistent disinterest.

2016 Dr. Marty Makary, and a co-author published an article stating that;

Medical Errors are the third leading cause of deaths in U.S. behind heart disease and cancer. And not an eye blinked in DC, and not an eye blinked in any of the fifty state capitals, and I did not understand that then, and 7 years later, I continue to not understand such ignorance. What will it take to make Decision Makers at Federal and State levels recognize a major problem?

Healthcare experts have been doing studies, writing articles, and a few books about the clearly recognizable, and long-standing problems within our Nation's HCDS, and yet, there has never been any attempt to create a thorough public debate, discussion, whatever regarding the well-documented problems within what I consider to be the greatest Social Responsibility of every Civilized Nation.

Healthcare Delivery System directly impacts the lives of every person from first breathe to last, plus those yet unborn, and that "System" has always been treated like an illegitimate child at a family reunion, and my assessment of that "System" is as follows.

Becoming a patient in any hospital in America is like shooting craps in Las Vegas, not everyone comes out a winner.

I have shot craps in Las Vegas, French Riviera, and other places, and that is an apt analogy. So, I am, and have long been, seeking someone who might help me understand; what will it take to finally elevate this critically important subject to a level of recognition, and consideration it should demand?

Introduction

This is a true, cautionary tale of how an argument between two middle-aged spouses, and the wife's regrettable response led to:

- The complete redirection of my life, and
- The exposure of one hospital medical staff, and Catholic administration's abandonment of all ethical and professional responsibility, and
- The incompetence of the Wisconsin Legislature, and its medical malpractice litigation civil court system, and more, far more.

"For Want of a Nail the Shoe was Lost" proverb came to mind as an apt reminder of how seemingly inconsequential events can initiate life-changing affects in the lives of unrelated individuals. And while the actions and events related throughout this complex story are true, the question must be asked; how can a story about events that took place over four decades ago be, not only interesting, but highly informative regarding current similar events?

The answer is based upon two facts; I have retained *all of the documents* related to this depiction of medical staff and Catholic administration malfeasance, and sadly, similar events have been taking place within hospital medical staffs, and throughout those agencies created to control such activities, during those past four decades. And it all begins when one middle-aged wife and mother made a simple mistake that would ultimately expose the unprofessional conduct of an entire religious-based health system and illustrate how truth can sometimes be stranger than fiction.

Madison Wisconsin, and its unique characteristics are renown; state capital, famous university and medical center, picturesque location between two sizable lakes, and a celebrated cultural center. Without Wisconsin winters the city population would explode. And for someone raised and educated in the

Deep South, the opportunity to practice my chosen profession as a member of a well-established surgical group within walking distance of the State Capital, and to be able to raise my young family while living in one of the most desirable residential areas of that great city was a dream come true. But that middle-aged woman who was only seeking non-urgent relief from me would set into motion a four-year process that would ultimately unravel my too-good-to-be-true dream world.

Little did I know that when that very pleasant wife and mother requested that I perform a simple oral surgical procedure of removing one upper molar tooth under outpatient general anesthesia as requested by her local dentist, my life would be dramatically re-directed, and our lives would be joined in an unplanned campaign that would lead to the exposure of the Dark Side of the medical profession, not only in Madison Wisconsin, but throughout the Nation. Sadly, the events of this story, while true, are merely a snap-shot of what has been a consistent pattern of hospital medical staff patient abuse throughout the history of our nation's medical profession, beginning with the creation of the first hospital in the Colonies in Philadelphia in the early 1740s, and culminating in the 2016 disclosure that Medical Errors are the 3rd leading cause of deaths in the U.S. behind heart disease and cancer. This story began when a middle-aged woman asked an oral surgeon to remove one upper molar tooth under general anesthesia, and thus both of us became active players in the future machinations of the medical malpractice litigation travesty in America.

Agnes was an average, middle-aged wife and mother when we not only entered, but invaded each other's life, and the Agnes I came to know would have never dreamed that her story might possess such long-lasting relevance.

While Agnes (now passed) and I would become the central focus of this demonstration of medical incompetence, and professional and legislative malfeasance, other participants would include:

- 2 ENT Surgeons who happened to be brothers.
- Hospital Medical Staff Executive Committee, and Administration.

- Joint Commission for the Accreditation of Hospitals (JCAH).
- Wisconsin Special Medical Malpractice Courts (an unbelievable farce).
- American Medical Association (AMA) abandonment of their ethical duty to patients.

Agnes' story exposes the unprofessional and unethical behavior of a religious-based hospital and medical clinic, medical staff leadership, and that religious-based hospital system Governance Board, Joint Commission, and the State of Wisconsin's ill-advised creation of a system of Special Medical Malpractice Courts. Other than that, Agnes was just an average, middle-aged wife and mother who was living and working in a small Wisconsin city.

Many will question the purpose in relating facts about a medical malpractice process that took place over 4 decades ago because of the time lapse, or perhaps with a desire not to look into the medical malpractice litigation system that has been an integral part of how questionable patient care cases have been reviewed for literally centuries. But the purpose of this rehashing of these events is to emphasize that no fundamental improvements in that doctor-favored process has ever taken place, and no one seems to care.

Agnes had a simple request; would I remove one upper molar tooth prior to her scheduled visit to see her original surgeon who supposedly had treated her fractured lower jaw several months previously. It was impossible for me to know that by fulfilling her request I would be ultimately facing one of those proverbial "forks in the road", and one path offered a life-changing outcome.

It is also important to understand how a four-month long, incompetent surgical treatment of a simple fracture of a person's lower jaw could lead to four years of biased medical peer review by a hospital and medical center's medical staff executive committee, and hospital administration, followed by the JCAH, and the short-lived Wisconsin State Medical Malpractice Panel system that was created as a response to the initial wave of the Mid-70s Medical Malpractice Crisis, and would soon prove to be a legislative nightmare. There is much that might be learned from a detailed revisit of this professional travesty, and far too few people interested in participating in such a re-visit.

I am a dentist. That said, I am a board-certified oral and maxillofacial surgeon and anesthesiologist, and I had joined the Kelly, Griffin, and Linn oral surgery group in Madison Wisconsin in 1966 after completing my 3-year oral surgery residency at the VA Hospital in Milwaukee. More importantly, the series of events depicted in this story would initiate the long-delayed process that has culminated in my becoming the author of multiple books on the Healthcare Delivery System (doctors & hospitals), and an expert regarding the efforts to improve the Quality of Care and Patient Safety aspects of that highly flawed "System". But, back to Agnes and I and how we became the David to the medical profession's Goliath.

One cannot practice surgery, even dental surgery, without coming face-to-face with less than desirable results provided by another surgeon. And becoming the second surgeon, tasked with attempting to correct a previous surgeon, or in this case, previous surgeons' surgical failure is one of the most unenviable positions imaginable.

The Dilemma: The 2nd surgeon must:

- Assess all of the details of the 1st surgeon's treatment plan, and surgery.
- Assess the patient's current post-operative condition.
- Formulate a treatment plan for the correction of the resultant post-surgical problem.
- Be given Current Treating Surgeon of Record authority by the first surgeon.
- Minimize professional shortcomings by the original surgeon (easier said than done), while adhering to the unwritten Code of Silence.

Surgical residencies and training programs do NOT include the dos and don'ts regarding the professional dilemma associated with second surgeon responsibilities. But what is inherently accepted as a second surgeon's professional responsibility is the Code of Silence. One may NEVER BREAK the CODE of SILENCE, regardless of the magnitude of the original surgeon's demonstrated incompetence. The second surgeon is *required* to speak to the patient, and other family members as though the original surgeon acted appropriately, but a few minor, unavoidable problems resulted. Unfortunately, attempts to accomplish such unethical behavior can prove to be difficult, if not impossible, as in Agnes' case. I would be able to successfully treat Agnes' long-standing surgical problem, but I could never erase her prior four-month ordeal from her memory.

Becoming the second surgeon is a surgeon's worst nightmare, and few surgeons make themselves readily available for such responsibility. I certainly did not seek to become the Madison Wisconsin second surgeon of choice regarding maxillofacial surgery cases, but subsequent events during the next several years would deem otherwise, because Agnes' care would prove to be just my beginning. But back to Agnes, and my fork-in-the-road.

Patient care need requiring a second surgeon to provide corrective care is a professional nightmare, and not just for the surgeons involved. Hospital medical staff leadership, and eventually hospital administration, and even Hospital Board of Governors should become involved, but in the real world of hospital governess, hospital leadership at every level do everything they can to be shielded from such disturbing matters. All of the above may be true, and it is; but one question remains.

Agnes' story goes behind the curtain, and into the dark portions of hospital medical staff, and administrations, and demonstrates the misguided, and unprofessional conduct of medical leadership that has been taking place in every hospital in America. It is a sad story that should cause people, and particularly healthcare decision-makers to take notice.

That is why Agnes' simple fracture of her lower jaw is important after 40 years. Agnes' current relevance is established due to the following facts: I retain all my patient care records, and the supporting documents of the events of her story, and Agnes' intrusion into my life that fateful day in 1979 initiated the arduous process that would lead to my ability to understand:

- Why our current Healthcare Delivery System (doctors & hospitals) is and has always been broken.
- How our current Healthcare Delivery System (doctors & hospitals) is, and has always been broken, and more importantly,
- How to begin to create a 21st century Healthcare Delivery System.

I consider the Healthcare Delivery System (HCDS) to be the most important *social responsibility* of every *civilized nation*. Why? That "system" directly impacts the lives of every living person, from first breath to last, plus those yet unborn. Yet the HCDS in every *civilized nation* is currently and has always been far less effective than it should be. Therefore, I am using Agnes' four-decade old story in an attempt to demonstrate that there has been NO fundamental improvement in our nation's HCDS during the past four decades, and no one seems to care. Agnes' story is very relevant today IF, and only if, it is given the critical consideration it deserves, so please join Agnes and I as we travel through the Dark Side of hospital medical staffs and administrations.

Agnes

Friday, November 2, 1979, and all was well in my life, or so I thought. I had been practicing oral surgery in a well-established group just 4 blocks from the State Capital, and the center of Madison Wisconsin since 1966. I had become board certified in early 1970, and in June of that year I, acting alone, had organized the first major surgical mini-residency of any surgical specialty in the Nation right there in Madison, and it had been a great success. I had demonstrated my ability to "think outside the box."

Mini-residencies are short, typically one-week, opportunities for practicing surgeons to gather and become qualified in expanding their personal scope of practice by observing new techniques of advanced surgical procedures. Our oral surgery specialty had been rapidly expanding to new methods for the surgical correction of jaw deformities since the mid-60s, and I had a strong desire to become adept at those new procedures.

A Journal of Oral Surgery Editorial in September 1969 written by the Chairman of an oral surgery residency suggested that "mini-residencies" were what our specialty needed to rapidly advance the ability for practicing surgeons to obtain the necessary experience to surgically treat patients with jaw deformities. That was my first exposure to the need for such programs that would enable practicing surgeons to gain such advanced expertise, and I instantly thought, "That is exactly what I need, and IF I am to get one, I need to create it for myself." And I did. What hubris!

I have to stop and shake my head now, but that snap decision, "that is what I need, and to get one, I need to create the first one for myself" declaration is exactly what took place in my mind. I began the first steps necessary to accomplish that first-of-a-kind feat a few days later. Such out of the box thinking proved to be possible in 1969, but I still look back and can only shake my head. I also told none of my senior colleagues of my plans, but I possess all of the documents necessary to support my audacious thinking that led to the first major surgical mini-residency in history.

To make a long story short, I was able to convince Edward Hinds, MD, DDS, Chairman of Oral Surgery, Un-Texas, Houston, to come to Madison in June 1970, and demonstrate advanced surgical procedures for myself, and multiple surgeons from 5 different states, but primarily from Wisconsin, and all participants said that week was one of their best experiences. I, of course, had obtained all of the patients necessary for the 5 days of surgery, and it was my responsibility to care for them after Dr. Hinds returned to Texas.

Parkland Hospital Oral Surgery Department in Dallas held the second major surgery mini-residency a few years later, and that program's sister residency program in Fort Worth held the third such mini-residency. Other oral surgery programs also soon began to hold such advanced training opportunities for practicing surgeons in other parts of the Nation. My initial game-changer event had provided the model for advanced surgical training, and I would participate in future mini-residency training, first at Parkland, and later at Fort Worth, as advancements in the correction of jaw deformities continued to escalate in our specialty well into the 1980s.

There is far more to the entire process of my creating the first major surgical mini-residency in the country, but I hope this brief summary will be sufficient. I continue to have all of the records of that historic event, and I was further gratified when I discovered that the American College of Ob/Gyn was lamenting their lack of, and great need for mini-residencies for their specialists in 2003 as I was doing research for my first book, FIRST, *DO NO HARM, THE CURE FOR MEDICAL MALPRCTICE,* published in 2004.

In October 1979, and only days before my first meeting with Agnes, I was in my second year as President of the Wisconsin Society of Oral Surgeons, and in that capacity, I had been meeting with the Secretary of the State Medical Society of Wisconsin regarding their providing administrative services for our members, as they did for several medical and non-medical societies in the state. In fact, the night I, and our Society President-Elect met with the Medical Society Secretary to finalize negotiations during dinner, he, the Medical Society Secretary, proceeded to choke on a bit of steak, and our President-Elect rapidly jumped up and clearly the obstruction using the Heimlich maneuver. He rapidly recovered, and we resumed business as if nothing had happened.

My wife and I had made plans to take our two sons, age 11, and 8 for two weeks travel that would include visits to 3 Hawaiian Islands during the Christmas and New Year Holidays. Life truly seemed too good to be true.

Agnes, my late morning patient, had been referred to our office for the removal of one upper molar tooth under general anesthesia by her local dentist. When I first met and spoke with both Agnes, and her husband, I was informed that she had been in an accident on June 28 in her hometown about 40 miles north of Madison, and that she was to see her treating doctor at the Dean Clinic that afternoon because she was still having great difficulty at her fracture site.

She had first been taken to St. Clare Hospital in her hometown of Baraboo, and diagnosed with two fractured ribs, and a fracture of her left lower jaw. She was treated for her rib fractures in that hospital, and then transferred to St. Mary's Hospital and Medical Center in Madison on July 1 for treatment of her jaw fracture. She told me that she had been having difficulties at her fracture site throughout the healing process during the past several months, and she was scheduled to see her primary surgeon that afternoon at his office at the Dean Clinic.

I told her that due to her history of a fractured lower jaw, and continuing problems at that fracture site, it would be necessary for my staff to take a Panorex x-ray so I could assess the current status of her injury. Agnes agreed, and the resultant x-ray demonstrated she had a major problem, and a necessary change in plans.

"Agnes, this x-ray shows that you are faced with a dilemma; you do need to have your upper tooth removed today because you are going to have to have further surgery at your fracture site; but I cannot use general anesthesia because I cannot put the necessary pressure on your lower jaw in order to open your mouth, therefore you are going to have to trust me that I can gently remove your upper tooth under local anesthetic."

A special note here: Panorex x-rays have become ordinary accessories, but their introduction in the 1960s provided a major advancement in the ability to obtain detail depictions of the bones and teeth of the jaws and mid-face not only for dentist, but also for those faced with the need to treat patients who had suffered facial trauma. Our oral surgery group had added the Panorex devise to our examination room in the late 1960s, and I had convinced the St. Mary's Hospital Chief of Radiology that they should include one in their expansion process of acquiring new equipment, and they did. The problem that would soon become evident was that those St. Mary's medical staff members who should have been using the benefits of that device choose to ignore it too often.

I was able to "gently remove" Agnes' upper molar tooth, and I gave her my Panorex x-ray to show to her treating doctor at the Dean Clinic later that afternoon, with the instructions that I wanted that x-ray returned to me for my records when he no longer needed it. After Agnes and her husband left my office, I called Dr. Tom, her Dean Clinic surgeon.

"Tom, Agnes just left my office. She and her husband were here so that I could extract her upper molar tooth that her dentist felt was beyond repair. I also took a Panorex x-ray, and it shows that she still has a non-union at her lower left mandibular fracture site. She is bringing my x-ray with her, but I will want it back at some time for my records, but only when you no longer need it.

"Ira, thanks for letting me know. We have been having difficulty with obtaining good healing at her fracture site, and I will call you again after I see her." Later that afternoon Dr. Tom called me.

"Ira, I see she does have a non-union at the fracture site. How would you treat such a complication?"

"Tom, there are multiple ways that might be used in treating this problem, but I would choose to use an external pin system called the Bi-Phase for this reason. Due to the long duration of the presence of a low-grade infection in the area due to the retained tooth in the line-of-fracture you cannot be sure that you can obtain normal healing at that fracture site with a simple open reduction, and the Bi-Phase pin fixation would still be in place if a bone graft would become necessary to finally obtain a firm union."

"Ira, we can't do that type of surgery. Would you treat her?"

"Yes, if that is O.K. with them. Have them return to my office now. I will wait and see them and make arrangements for admitting her to surgery. But Tom, I will need to admit her to Methodist Hospital because their OR nurses are more accustomed to assisting me in my major surgery cases, including Bi-Phase system, and I hope you understand.

"Ira, I do, and that is fine with me, but will you let me know when she is admitted for surgery?"

"Yes, I will give you a call the day she is admitted to Methodist."

Agnes and her husband returned to my office that afternoon, and due to the late hour, I asked that she return on Monday the 5th so that I could remove her lower molar tooth that had been left in the line of fracture for the past 4 months, and had been the source of her constant state of infection, and the cause of her failure to achieve normal healing. I also started her on antibiotics.

Incompetence is defined as, lacking qualification or ability, or not legally qualified. Agnes's story documents the incompetence of two board certified ENT surgeons, who happened to be brothers, and due to their failure to remove the lower molar tooth in the line of her fracture that would be the source of her post-operative problems for four months, and including two hospitalizations, and two surgeries. Doctors Dumb and Dumber would demonstrate complete incompetence, and the St. Mary's Hospital medical staff and administration, including the Board of Governors, would elevate their level of incompetence, and make it that hospital's accepted standard of care for future treatment of mandibular fractures. Agnes would not be the only person who would suffer the consequences of becoming a patient in St. Mary's Hospital for the treatment of lower jaw injuries, but Agnes's story, and the details of her story must come first.

Bi-Phase system of external pin fixation was created by Dr. Joe Hall Morris at the University of Tennessee in Memphis, and he was one of my early mentors there during my dental student years, and a close friend later. The Bi-Phase pin system became widely used in all parts of the world due to its relatively ease of use, and source of firm fixation. I would use that system on several of my patients when the need arose.

Methodist Hospital was the smallest of the three private hospitals in Madison at that time and located only a block from our oral surgery clinic. When I had my first thoughts about creating the first major surgical mini residency in the entire history of surgery in America in 1970, I realized that I needed three key elements to make such an event possible.

First, I would need a dual-degree MD/DDS surgeon to conduct the event and provide all of the surgery to the patients. I went to the State Medical Board located a few short blocks from our clinic and described Dr. Edward Hines' impressive credentials as Chairman of Oral Surgery at the University of Texas in Houston, and also as the world-wide U.S. Air Force oral surgery consultant. Their response was, "Yes, there would be no question but that he would be provided with a temporary license to practice medicine and surgery in Wisconsin." One down, and two to go.

I next met with Bill Johnson, Methodist Hospital Administrator and described my intent. Bill said, "Yes", they would provide an OR for each morning, and a lecture room for the afternoon, and lunch for all attendees, and he was excited to be a part of such an event. Two down, and now Dr. Hinds would be the deciding factor. Fortunately, he too would agree, and the rest became history nine years before Agnes entered my life.

Also, that 1970 event initiated Bill Johnson, and the Methodist Hospital Board, and Medical Executive Committee to decide to create a Dental Department and allow the Chairman of that Department to become a member of the Medical Staff Executive Committee. But the unspoken reason for such a major departure in the structure of hospital medical staffs was obvious; it was to increase patient care use, and profitability by providing the local dentists with a hospital that would welcome them. I would serve as Chairman of the Dental Department for two two-year terms during the 1970s. But back to Agnes' story.

Agnes, and her husband, were the last patients I saw on that 5th of November so long ago, and I called my wife and told her I would be somewhat late arriving home that evening as I had another stop to make. I needed to know the details of Agnes' care for those past four months, and why, and how she could appear in my office with an infected, and non-healed lower jaw fracture four months after her initial treatment, and the answers to my questions could only be found in her medical records at St. Mary's Hospital.

Drs. Tom and Tim

My delay going home was due to my desire and need to see Agnes' medical records at St. Mary's Hospital and Medical Center, but I was not prepared for what I saw and read. I did have Courtesy Medical Staff privileges at St. Mary's and at Madison General Hospital, and therefore I felt that as her new treating surgeon I had a right to examine her record.

Dr. Tom Donovan, a board-certified ENT surgeon practicing at the Dean Clinic was assigned to treat her injury upon her admission to that hospital, and it must be noted here that upon her first admission she had several x-rays taken, including a Panorex x-ray that included a detail view of both jaws and her mid-face. This would be the only adequate x-ray taken of her original jaw injury, and future jaw complications during the 4 long months under the care of two board certified ENT surgeons.

Upon arrival at St. Mary's, I first visited the Radiology Department and examined her x-ray files. What I discovered was shocking to me. Agnes had had several x-rays taken on her first day admission, including the excellent Panorex x-ray that clearly demonstrated her pre-operative status at the fracture site. But there were NO additional Panorex x-rays ever taken post-operative even though she had had two hospital admissions, and in-house stays for almost two weeks each. Thus, my Panorex x-ray taken on November 2, four months after her first hospital admission was the ONLY ADEQUATE POST-OPERATIVE X-RAY ever taken. Sadly, there was more to come.

Agnes' medical records demonstrated incompetence of the highest order. Agnes was operated on for correction of her jaw fracture on July 3 by Dr. Tom and assisted by his brother Dr. Tim. Her operation consisted of a surgical open reduction, and fixation of her lower jaw to her upper jaw by arch bars, and intermaxillary wires. The open reduction consisted of a surgical incision in the skin of her upper neck for access to the inferior border of her lower jaw, and the fracture site. Holes were drilled into the lower border of both fragments at the fracture site, and wire ligatures were used to pull the two fragments into close proximity. The surgical wound was closed, and her lower jaw was fixed to her upper jaw by wires connecting the upper and lower arch bars. Everything was done in a customary manner for open reduction of a lower jaw fracture—EXCEPT—one must remove the tooth in the line of fracture or else post-operative infection will prevent normal healing, and that simple procedure was never done, thus creating the source of her future 4-months of post-operative Infection.

Unfortunately, the key to all of Agnes', and my future problems, was that both medically trained surgeons lacked the fundamental understanding that the *lower tooth in the line of fracture must be removed, or it will be the source of infection, and non-healing of the fracture.* Everything that was to follow in Agnes', and her family's life, and ultimately into my life, would stem from that simple, and inexcusable failure. Agnes had two surgeons attempting to provide her with medical care that was beyond their collective understanding, and all parties involved, then, and later, would pay an enormous price for their stupidity. But July 3rd was only the beginning. The rest of Agnes' four months of care provided by those two surgeons should classify them as Doctors Dumb and Dumber because *everything,* they would do in those coming months would be wrong.

Dr. Tom's DISCHARGE SUMMARY provides details of Act 1 in Agnes' tragic story.

Admitted:	7-1-79
Discharged:	7-13-79

This patient is a white female who enters St. Mary's with a history of facial trauma, transferred down from St. Clair's Hospital. She has an obvious mandible fracture. She was taken to the Operation Room where she had an open reduction of her mandibular fracture on 7-3-79. Post operation there was some complication with some draining from her left neck wound. This drainage has become minimal amount at the present time. Her condition on discharge is stable and satisfactory.

FINAL DIAGNOSIS:	*Facial trauma with a fracture of the mandible on the left.*
OPERATIONS:	*Open reduction, intramaxillary fixation, left mandibular fracture.*
COMPLICATIONS:	*NONE*

IF the tooth in the line of fracture had been removed, as it should have been, she would have been discharged from the hospital the day after surgery, or no later than two days after surgery, AND with NO DRAINAGE to the neck incision. Instead, Agnes spent 13 days in the hospital, and was discharged with obvious clinical evidence of an infection with a "foul odor" six days after surgery. And that infection would continue for four months, another hospitalization, and another trip to the Operating Room because two board certified surgeons didn't know what they didn't know.

Dr. Tom's Discharge Summary note:

COMPLICATIONS: *NONE demonstrates the height of stupidity and incompetence.*

July 20 (*7 days after discharge*) *Agnes was seen by Dr. Tom in the Dean Clinic, and he noted in her medical record, "some drainage", but no post-operative x-ray taken.*

July 23 Agnes returned to Dean Clinic, and Dr. Tom noted, "some drainage". Still no post-operative x-ray.

July 29 As Agnes would relate her story to me because, as her treating surgeon I had a need to know the details of her history with her current problem; she was lying in bed one morning, and as she rolled over, she heard, and felt, a crack at her fracture site. She called the Dean Clinic and was told that Dr. Tom was not available, but Dr. Tim would be able to see her the next day.

July 30 Agnes returned to the Dean Clinic. When she arrived at the Dean Clinic additional x-rays of her fracture site were taken, but that clinic only had the ability to attempt to obtain x-rays using large flat plates, and the multiple x-rays taken that day were very inadequate for the need.

Dr. Tim noted in her Clinic record, "Patient has infection", and she was admitted to the hospital "for IV antibiotics", and he proceeded to have Agnes re-admitted to St. Mary's with obvious signs of infection at the wound site in her neck. Agnes was admitted into a room with another patient, and no admission Panorex x-ray was ordered. Dr. Tim had broken all hospital protocol by not admitting Agnes, with an obvious infection, into Isolation. Instead, Agnes was instructed to roll her IV stand down the hallway to a public restroom and apply hot moist compresses to her neck area periodically each day.

Agnes' second hospitalization reads like something out of a comic book. Dr. Tim admitted her on July 30, just 17 days after she had been discharged by Dr. Tom with "NO COMPLICATIONS". She was placed on antibiotics, and hot moist compresses, but provided NO direct treatment or consideration for the source of her infection. Dt. Tim took her to the Operating Room and provided "Re-alignment of Mandibular Fracture", and the total procedure took 35 min. But there was no mention of the tooth in the line of fracture. She was discharged on August 10.

> **_August 16_** Dr. Tom noted, "shifting of occlusion" in her medical record.
>
> **_August 28_** Dr. Tom noted, "arch bars removed", leaving Agnes with no mandibular fixation, and an infected, non-union at the fracture site.
>
> **_September 19_** Dr. Tom noted, "Looks good".
>
> **_October 17_** Dr. Tom noted, "more drainage".
>
> **_November 5_** I received the following letter from Agnes' local dentist, Dr. Arnold Utzinger:

> Dear Dr. Williams,
>
> First saw Mrs. Woodbury 8-20-79. Was on the 20th day of intermax. fixation following the second surgical reduction of lower left area.
>
> The first operation was July 3, and had bilateral reduction at that time.

> *She said the need for a second surgery was that her "bite was shifting". I assume that meant she had a non-union at that time and so was retreated.*
>
> *I then saw her again on 10-19-79. Had external submand. drainage & had been started on Keflex by Dr. Donovan. (Had fixation removed about Sept. 10). At this appt. (10-19) we referred her to your office. (Note: typical abbreviations of words in short note)*
>
> *Sincerely,*
> **Dr. Utzinger**

Agnes' summary includes: two admissions totaling 25 days, 1 pre-operative Panorex x-ray, lots of antibiotics, and NO adequate post-operative x-ray., plus being admitted with an obvious infection, and no isolation protocol. And at some point-in-time after her August 10 discharge from St. Mary's she had her arch bars and intermaxillary fixation removed, although there had been NO healing at the fracture site.

I was totally dismayed when I left St. Mary's that night and drove home. I could not fathom such surgical and intellectual stupidity. After the first admission Panorex x-ray those two board certified surgeons had done everything wrong, and Agnes had been their unwilling victim.

Her first two months, July, and August were the first acts in a tragic play that would run for the best part of four years, and Agnes and I had no clue as to what lay ahead. But one thing needs to be made clear here and repeated later; during all of my activities in seeking to help her and her husband receive some level of compensation for all of the pain and suffering she endured, no one on the other side of this issue ever asked, "How is the patient doing!" As the details unfold, once I asked that Agnes' care at Dean Clinic and St. Mary's Hospital and Medical Center be reviewed the issue became adversarial, and Agnes became their enemy.

But first, I had to surgically correct Agnes' on-going problem, and get her lower jaw where healing could begin to take place.

My Turn

Agnes was admitted to Methodist Hospital on November 12, and I called Dr. Tom and told him she was scheduled for surgery the next morning. Dr. Tom visited Agnes in her room that night and told her how sorry he was for the difficulties she had suffered, but she needed to know that she had first presented herself to him with one of the most difficult mandibular fractures he had ever seen, and that sometimes in dealing with extreme trauma complications do occur. And I tend to agree with Dr. Tom that Agnes' initial fracture *may have been* one of the most extreme traumatic injuries to the lover jaw that he had seen, but her initial fracture was, in fact, a very simple fracture of her mandible with a tooth in the line of fracture, and no displacement of the fragments.

A first-year oral surgery resident could have successfully treated Agnes' initial injury, and without difficulty, but that first-year resident would have removed that tooth in the line of fracture. I had also called him after the surgery the next day, and told him all had gone well, and that I was satisfied with what had been accomplished.

November 13, 1979, Agnes was taken to the Methodist Hospital Operation Room, and I performed an open reduction basically similar to the one performed by Dr. Tom, and assisted by Dr. Tim on July 3, except I had removed the offending tooth in the line of fracture the previous week, and finally allowed normal healing to begin to take place.

Due to her long-standing infection at the fracture site during the past several months there was some uncertainty that so much normal bone may have deteriorated, thus preventing a firm healing to take place between the fragments, and thereby necessitating a bone graft in the area. Therefore, I used the Bi-Phase system of two large self-tapping screws placed in the distal fragment, and two additional screws placed in the proximal fragment, and those screws were connected by a solid bar fashioned out of acrylic (denture material). While unsightly, that system of four screws locked together by that bar provided the necessary fixation, and could remain in place IF evidence of firm, normal healing at the fracture site did not take place in the coming weeks.

Agnes was discharged from Methodist Hospital on the 17th, and subsequent follow-up visits showed no post-operative problems, except for one. November 26 Agnes told me that on November 20 she had slipped and received a blow to the head, but no damage to the fracture site, or external fixation. The Bi-Phase system is so solid that it might even be possible to lift someone off their feet, and not dislodge the screws.

On January 19, 1980, I ascertained that clinical healing had taken place, and all fixation, bar, screws, and arch bars were removed. Agnes had endured 6 1/2 months of misery for a process that should have taken only six weeks. I continued to see Agnes, but on a very limited basis for there was no need.

March 15 Agnes was seen in my office, and she had a small, firm, mobile mass at her fracture site in the soft tissue beneath her skin that was presumed to be of no concern, but just scar tissue due to her long-standing, and consistent infection in the area.

July 9 Agnes was seen for the last time in my office. I performed a simple smoothing of the alveolar ridge in the area of the fracture and performed a root canal on her lower right cuspid incisor under local anesthesia. Agnes had become a much more relaxed patient by then, but she and I didn't even talk about past events. So, I can relate the events of a not-so-simple open reduction of a mandibular fracture in two pages simply because I took the precaution of removing the tooth in the line of fracture.

But neither Agnes or her husband had the slightest indication of how I had initiated a medical peer review process regarding her highly questionable care within the St. Mary's Hospital and Medical Center Medical Staff, and I had no intention of informing them of a process that I considered to be limited to myself and St. Mary's medical peer review system.

I had successfully corrected Agnes' surgical problem, but that would prove to be the easy part of her ordeal. I was left on the horns of a dilemma; my professional responsibility to Agnes, St. Mary's Hospital and Medical Center as a member of its medical staff, and to myself. The easiest thing to do was to do what is almost always done in such cases, say NOTHING. But I felt that the St. Mary's Medical Staff leadership had to be told of the grossly negligent manner in which Agnes had received treatment from two of their surgeons for a period of four months, and with such total disregard for proper professional responsibilities.

My efforts to seek a process for how to fulfill my ethical responsibility to the hospital medical staff, while attempting to maintain my professional integrity would begin prior to completion of Agnes' healing process, and with her original two surgeons. That process would ultimately expose the Dark Side of Medical Peer Review at St. Mary's Hospital and Medical Center, and in Madison Wisconsin.

History of Healthcare

Take a small roast, add some carrots, small onions, and small potatoes, and bake in an oven, and you would have a meal that provides all the excitement of kissing one's sister. Ask a qualified cook to take the same ingredients, and add species and condiments, and invited guests would declare it to be a wonderful meal. Spices are the key to great cooking.

History provides spices to one's intellect.
Historical Snapshots

I was born 68 years after the end of the Civil War, and 22 years later, as an Air Force navigator, I was flying with a pilot at 50,000 feet in the precursor of the U-2, and our mission would have been to deliver tactical atomic bombs if WWIII had begun during the Cold War at that time.

Beethoven died the year Andrew Jackson was elected to become the 7th President of the United States, and ten years later a very young Victoria became Queen of England.

Those who ignore history never realized they have chosen to ignore the spices of their intellect. I can't imagine a life devoid of the desire to include historical context in my thoughts. Therefore, this documentary exposure of the dark side of one Catholic Hospital's entire medical staff leadership, and one Catholic Healthcare System's governing board's choice to ignore all ethical and professional responsibilities in their efforts to deny grossly negligent patient care deserves to be accepted as historically relevant fact.

Medical Peer Review

There are three "systems" with the potential to review questionable patient care. I hate the term medical malpractice because it assumes a negative. Not all medical complications are malpractice, therefore my preference for the term questionable patient care.

Medical peer review is the only one of those three "systems" where doctors are, or can be, and should be, in complete control of the process. But true, effective, medical peer review, equally fair to both doctor and patient is as rare as snow fall in New Orleans (my daddy was born and raised in Louisiana, and in 1962 I would obtain a Louisiana Dental License).

The problem is, and has always been, that doctors do not know how to fairly judge the questionable patient care by other doctors. But doctors know all too well the AMA edict, Code of Silence. Furthermore, doctors know that IF they were to participate in medical peer review of another doctor, that would mean that they too might face such patient care review, and again, doctors know that they do not know how to fairly judge the questionable patient care of each other, and they have NO desire to learn how to judge their fellow practitioners.

That said, I felt I had a responsibility to share my concerns, and I felt my first step must be in meeting with her original two surgeons and share my concerns. Dr. Tom had already demonstrated contrition both to me and to Agnes when he met with her at Methodist Hospital the evening prior to her surgery to correct his, and his brother's failures.

December 3, 1979, I called the ENT office at Dean Clinic, and arranged to meet with both surgeons at their office at the end of the day. Dr. Dibble, the senior and 3rd member of the Dean Clinic ENT Department was also present. Needless to say, the meeting was less than cordial. I began by saying that, as a member of St. Mary's medical staff I felt I had a responsibility to share my concerns for her previous care with someone on the hospital medical staff. The response by the two doctors differed dramatically.

It is difficult to capture all that is said when four people, not all on the same page, are speaking (yes, Dr. Dibble expressed his views that all had gone well during Agnes' treatment at both the Dean Clinic and St. Mary's Hospital). I, of course, felt that I was walking on thin ice, when everyone in the room knew all that had taken place during the past 5 months regarding Agnes' fractured jaw. I was finally asked.

Ira, what do you want to do? I feel I have a responsibility to share my concerns with someone on the Medical Staff who has a need to know when questionable patient care takes place. But I did not want to speak to anyone on the Medical Staff without first sharing my concerns with both of you. (Speaking to Dr. Tom and Dr. Tim)

Dr. Tim. Ira, I suppose you have been sharing your concerns with Agnes.

Absolutely not! I have said nothing about my concerns to either Agnes or her husband, and I have no intention to do so in the future. My concerns are only a matter for the Hospital Medical Staff.

Dr. Tim. Ira, you can speak to anyone on the Medical Staff you want to because we did nothing wrong.

Dr. Tim's forceful declaration said what I needed to be told. I had not wanted to say anything about Agnes' care to anyone before I spoke with her original two surgeons, and as uncomfortable as it had been, I had checked that off my list, and now felt free to seek to initiate a peer review process within that Hospital's Medical Staff. That is how I thought the process should be conducted.

Dr. Tim had seen Agnes at Dean Clinic in late July after she had experienced the "cracking" sound at her fracture site and was being seen on an emergency basis. He had diagnosed her as having an infection and had admitted her into St. Mary's without Isolation Protocol, and into a room with a roommate, and had her expose her active infection to that roommate, and other patients, and members of the public as she walked the corridor in her efforts to apply hot, moist compresses to her active, infected drainage. Furthermore, he had subjected Agnes to another general anesthetic while he "realigned her intermaxillary fixation", and ignored the source of her infection, the tooth in the line of fracture. Dr. Tim was unbelievable in my view, but at least I had taken the first, and in my opinion, the proper step in initiating a peer review process regarding Agnes' highly questionable care by first speaking with her initial surgeons.

St. Mary's Hospital and Medical Center not only had a Medical Staff Leadership system, but also a Medical Director. I called and spoke with Dr. Vinograd, the Medical Director, the next day, and he said he would get back with me. Three days later he called me and said that I was to contact Dr. Baranowski. I called him, and he suggested that we meet at a private club in downtown Madison next week.

December 12, 1979, I met with Dr. Baranowski in the private club's bar and lounge, and I found him to be very cordial, and seemingly interested in how I might suggest an effective process for review of Agnes' care at St. Mary's. I said that there were both ENT and Oral Surgery training programs at both the University of Iowa, and University of Minnesota Hospitals, and that I would provide copies of my Panorex x-ray taken on the first day I saw her in my office along with a detail letter of my treatment for her injury.

He said that that was a great idea, and that he would recommend that they send copies of all of their records and x-rays to all four training programs, so would I please provide them with four copies of my Panorex x-ray, and letter. I said I would and left our brief meeting with the false hope that they would actually follow through, and five days later I delivered the requested x-rays and my letter to him.

I had also become aware that there was a lot of "cocktail talk" taking place within the medical community, and I called Dr. Tim. He confirmed that he had been discussing Agnes' case with the University of Wisconsin Chairman of the ENT Department, and various Plastic Surgeons in the area, and that all had agreed that he and his brother had "done nothing wrong." Thus ended the peer review process through the Holidays of 1979, and I and my family spent the Holidays happily visiting three Hawaiian Islands, while I left my concerns for Agnes' care and medical peer review in Madison. Little did I know what the New Year would bring.

Remember, I said *effective peer review, fair to both doctor and patient,* and *leaves doctors in control.* And because I had provided copies of my initial Panorex x-ray demonstrating Agnes' non-union, and the offending tooth in the line of fracture after two hospitalizations, two surgeries, and four months of questionable care, I assumed I would only take part in their peer review process if asked. Unfortunately, St. Mary's Medical Staff process of peer review would be a peer review disgrace, and also without any thought of the patient.

On January 6, 1980, I called Dr. Baranowski and was told that he was to meet with the Medical Director, and Chief of the Medical Staff. What ultimately transpired should be seen as highly predictable; St. Mary's Medical Staff leaders had NO intention of requesting a review of Agnes' care at their hospital by even one of the four potential University Residency Programs in Iowa or Minnesota, therefore I was later to learn the following.

A special meeting of the surgery patient review committee was held at 6:00 p.m. on January 29, 1980. Present were Drs. Baranowski, Bernsten, Bernhardt, Colburn, S. T. Donovan, T.J. Donovan, Dibble, Engeler, Hetsko, Hoffman, Licklider, Pellegrino, Shannahan, Vinograd, Wenger, and Woodford.

The meeting was called to review the treatment rendered to Agnes Woodbury, Chart #597889 at the request of Ira E. Williams, D.D.S. Attached is a communication from Dr. Williams and a file note dated December 4, 1979, from "St. Mary's Medical Director". Mrs. Woodbury, a 41-year-old female, was transferred from Baraboo Hospital after a 3-day hospitalization, for treatment of mandibular fracture. The patient was treated with open reduction internal fixation of fracture and arch bar immobilization. The fracture extended through a tooth but did not fracture either the root or the common tooth. The patient subsequently developed drainage from the fracture site and was treated with antibiotics. The drainage persisted requiring a second admission approximately 4 weeks later. The patient was admitted and treated with intravenous antibiotics and the patient's drainage ceased. The patient was seen by Dr. Williams at the patient's dentist's request for another problem. The patient was admitted to Methodist Hospital where the tooth was extracted (not true) and an external fixation device applied. Dr. Williams raised several points which he felt represented inappropriate treatment. He met with Drs. Donovan and Dibble, at the Dean Clinic and questioned the lack of initial x-rays at hospital. It was pointed out that the initial x-rays were taken in Baraboo and were considered adequate. The question of whether the tooth involved at the fracture line should have been extracted initially was raised. It was felt by the treating surgeon that the tooth was the only anchor posterior to the fracture line and extraction was not indicated at that time. When the patient was re-hospitalized, again the question of x-rays not being available was raised. Apparently, the x-rays had been taken at the Dean Clinic on the day of admission. Dr. Williams questioned the adequacy of the postoperative x-rays. Dr. Colburn stated that the frontal projection and two obliques were the standard views used for mandibular fractures prior to having Panorex available and that these in his opinion were adequate. The wound and skin care were questioned as was the absence of culture reports. (Two culture reports were available from the clinic.)

Dr. Bernsten commented on the care provided by Mrs. Woodbury and stated that he felt the drainage was a complication of treatment rather than representing inadequate treatment. Infection following open reduction of mandibular fractures and subsequent non-union was a well-recognized complication. He did not feel that extraction of the tooth was indicated initially. He also pointed out that in these cases delayed extraction of the tooth usually led to resolution of the infection and prompt healing.

After much discussion it was adjudged that Dr. Williams' criticisms did not warrant duplication of the charts and having the information sent to the Department of Otolaryngology and Oral Surgery at the Universities of Iowa and Minnesota. It was felt unanimously by the committee that the differences were ones of judgment and not inadequacy.

A letter will be written to this affect informing Dr. Williams of the committee's decision.

Signed: Dr. Baranowski, Chairman, Surgery Patient Review Committee.

[**My note:** *Welcome to the real world of medical peer review. Sixteen doctors, "after much discussion" proceeded to justify gross, negligent patient care at every point of four months of negligent care, and everyone left that meeting feeling satisfied. What they failed to understand was that that report created a new standard of care for future mandibular fracture open reductions at that hospital to the lowest possible level conceivable, and all in the name of the Code of Silence. Unfortunately, those medical experts left that room thinking they had just put an end to the Peer Review of Agnes' negligent care at that Hospital and Medical Center, but their assumption would soon be proven otherwise.*]

On January 31, 1980, I received the following letter from Dr. Baranowski, Chairman of the Surgery Patient Review Committee.

> Dear Dr. Williams,
>
> The Surgery Patient Review Committee of St. Mary's Hospital Medical Center met on January 29, 1980. The purpose of the meeting was to review the treatment afforded Agnes Woodbury at St. Mary's in July and August of 1979.

After review of the patient's chart and x-rays and much discussion and deliberation, it was felt that the questions raised by you in your letter of December 15, 1979, represented differences in judgement rather than inadequate or inappropriate treatment.

Signed, Dr. Baranowski, Chairman, Surgery Patient Review Committee

Differences in judgement? I could only wonder how a committee of physicians could possibly review the multiple facts of surgical negligence clearly apparent in her hospital records and demonstrated so clearly in my Panorex x-ray (the only adequate post-operative x-ray ever taken in 4 months of treatment) and conclude there was merely "a difference of judgement".

I could only *assume* that "they" *assumed* the Surgery Patient Review process had been completed at the close of the Review Committee's meeting. WRONG!

Medical Peer Review Continues

February 1, I called Dr. Baranowski's office, and spoke with his nurse after lunch. He was to call me after seeing his last patient, but he never called, therefore I wrote the following letter that day.

> *Stephen Dudiak, M.D.*
> Chief of Staff
> St. Mary's Hospital
> Madison, Wisconsin
>
> Dear Dr. Dudiak,
>
> I am writing to you regarding Mrs. Agnes Woodbury of Baraboo, Wisconsin.
>
> Mrs. Woodbury was a patient at St. Mary's with admissions on July 1, 1979, and July 30, 1979.
>
> Mrs. Woodbury's care was transferred to me voluntarily on November 2, 1979, by her then attending physicians who had treated her during her two previous admissions.
>
> On December 3, 1979, I met with the previous physicians to discuss my concerns for aspects of the care they had rendered to Mrs. Woodbury.
>
> It was agreed at that time by <u>all</u> parties present that I would approach the St. Mary's Medical Director. He was to direct me to the committee chairman of his choice for further discussions.
>
> I met with Walter O. Baranowski, M.D., Chairman of the Surgery Patient Review Committee on December 13, 1979.
>
> To date, I have <u>no</u> information that the care rendered Mrs. Woodbury during her two admissions of July 1979 has been reviewed.
>
> I find this delay difficult to comprehend.

> As a member of your staff (Courtesy) and as Mrs. Woodbury's present primary care physician regarding these matters, I do request some acknowledgement of my concerns—soon.
>
> I would appreciate hearing from you as soon as possible as to my original request; does the care rendered Mrs. Woodbury during the period July 1, 1979, to November 2, 1979, meet the standard of care of St. Mary's hospital?
>
> Sincerely,
> **Ira E. Williams, D.D.S.**

February 4, I called the Chief of Staff office and requested minutes of the Surgery Patient Review Committee meeting I was told had taken place.

> February 6, 1980
>
> **Ira E. Williams, D.D.S.**
> 416 W. Mifflin Street
> Madison, WI 53703
>
> Dear Dr. Williams,
>
> Replying to your telephone request of February 4, 1980, minutes and lists of attendees of meetings of the departmental and patient review committees of our medical staff are open and available for review. Although they are not secret, they are regarded as private documents since they reflect the inner workings of the staff and often deal with sensitive and potentially sensitive issues. It is, therefore, hospital policy that copies are not distributed. Minutes and rosters are made available for review by staff members in the Medical Staff Office, room 1206. Mrs. Rozinski, my secretary, who is in charge of these records, will be pleased to locate the minutes of the January 29 meeting for your perusal. She is there from 7:00 a.m. to 3:30 p.m. Monday through Friday. The office is closed on weekends and holidays.
>
> I understand that you are to meet with Dr. Dudiak, our Chief of Staff, this evening. If there are still some unresolved questions in your mind, I would suggest in the interest of everyone's time that you meet with Dr. Dudiak, Dr. Baranowskii, Dr. Pellegrino who our Chief of Surgery is, and myself in a single meeting in order to clear the air of questions on both sides. I will be pleased to make

> *the appropriate arrangements as soon as you notify me of your availability.*
>
> *As you know, St. Mary's Hospital Medical Center is dedicated to adherence to the highest standards of quality of medical care that we can provide. The St. Mary's Medical Staff has, according to its Bylaws, established the administrative mechanisms which enable it to investigate thoroughly by peer examination any case in which a significant issue is raised. By calling this matter into question you have clearly discharged your obligations to both the patient and this hospital and have made it possible for us, through the use of these established peer review procedures, to assure ourselves that in this instance the outcome, though not a desirable one, was not due to any diagnostic or therapeutic impropriety.*
>
> *Sincerely yours,*
>
> **S.H. Vinograd, M.D.,**
> Medical Director

This letter was my chance to ignore the facts of Agnes' four months of grossly negligent care provided by two board-certified surgeons and adhere to the Code of Silence. I knew full well that I was following a path seldom traveled, and there would be a price I would have to pay IF I continued down that path, yet I also knew that what I did next would define myself, to myself, and I was not willing to "sell my soul" to the Code of Silence. The following events in this process would change my life forever, and I have never regretted my choice.

February 7, I finally was given an opportunity to visit the Medical Director's office and see the January 29 Surgery Patient Review Committee report. When I entered the office Dr. Vinograd was standing in the doorway to his office, and he instantly moved toward me, but with no offer of a welcoming hand.

Are you a troublemaker?

No. That is not my intention, but I do believe Mrs. Woodbury's care during her four months of treatment by two of your surgeons demanded review. I was asked to provide 4 Panorex x-rays of what I consider to be the first adequate post-operative x-ray ever taken following her initial surgery on July 3, and her second hospitalization later that month.

Here is the Committee report, and you can read it here. (After reading the report) May I have a copy of the report. No.

> February 8, 1980
>
> **Ernest A. Pellegrino, M.D.**
> Chief of Surgery
> St. Mary's Hospital
> Madison, Wisconsin
>
> Dear Dr. Pellegrino,
>
> *I am writing to you in regard to Mrs. Woodbury of Baraboo, Wisconsin. Mrs. Woodbury was a patient at St. Mary's Hospital in July 1979 and again in August 1979. Mrs. Woodbury's care was voluntarily transferred to me in November 1979.*
>
> *As a member in good standing (courtesy) of the St. Mary's Hospital staff and being appointed to the Department of Surgery I am writing you to request that the Executive Committee respond to me in writing regarding Mrs. Woodbury's care from July 1, 1979, to November 2, 1979.*
>
> *I am aware that this matter was reviewed by the Surgery Patient Review Committee on January 29, 1980. Dr. Baranowski was kind enough to write me regarding their findings. And this request is <u>not</u> meant to question the findings of that committee.*
>
> *However, according to your By-laws, Article VI, Section III, A, (2) the Executive Committee will receive and act upon reports of the Medical Staff and hospital committees as designated.*
>
> *I feel very strongly the interests of my patient, and myself will best be served if the Executive Committee will reply to my request that Mrs. Woodbury's treatment does or does not meet the standard of care for St. Mary's Hospital.*
>
> *Sincerely,*
> **Ira E. Williams, D.D.S.**

> February 15, 1980
>
> **Stephen Dudiak, M.D.**
> Chief of Staff
> St. Mary's Hospital
> Madison, WI 53715
>
> Dear Dr. Dudiak,
>
> After review of the minutes of the Surgery Patient Review Committee of St. Mary's Hospital and much deliberation, I am unable to accept the findings of that committee on January 29, 1980.
>
> I request that the treatment rendered Mrs. Woodbury between July 1, 1979, and November 2, 1979, remain open to further review.
>
> Sincerely,
> **Ira E. Williams, D.D.S.**

(With that letter the barnyard excrement [I cleaned that up] hit the fan!)

> February 21, 1980
>
> **Ira E. Williams, D.D.S.**
> 416 W. Mifflin Street
> Madison WI 53703
>
> Dear Dr. Williams,
>
> During its last meeting, held on Monday, February 18, 1980, the Executive Committee of the St. Mary's Hospital Medical Staff examined the issues concerning the case of Mrs. Agnes Woodbury. The committee reviewed the minutes of the special meeting of the Surgery Patient Review Committee and your letters to Dr. Dudiak and Dr. Pellegrino. In view of your

expression of disagreement with the findings of the Surgery Patient Review Committee and your request that the matter remain open to further review, no action was taken pending receipt of further information from you outlining the nature of your disagreement.

It is, therefore, requested that you submit to the Executive Committee prior to its next meeting on March 17, 1980, a letter stating specifically your reasons for disagreeing with the treatment rendered to Mrs. Woodbury by her attending physicians at this hospital in July and August of 1979. Moreover, the reasons for your reservations concerning the proceedings of the January 29, 1980, Surgery Patient Review Committee meeting with respect to this matter should be stated specifically, as well. In addition, your presence will be required during the discussion of this agenda item at the next Executive Committee meeting. This will take place at 6:30 p.m. on Monday, March 17, 1980, in Dining Room A, just adjacent to the hospital cafeteria on the A level.

The Executive Committee will make its judgement of an appropriate course of action based upon the written and verbal commentary which you provide together with all other evidence available to it.

Sincerely,
Stephen Dudiak, M.D.,
Chief of Staff

(Being a member of the St. Mary's Medical Staff I received copies by mail like the following.)

St. Mary's Hospital Medical Center
MEDICAL STAFF NEWSLETTER,
February 1980

Chief of Staff ANNUAL REPORT

The Annual Report of the Chief of Staff was presented by Dr. Dudiak at the Annual Staff Meeting held on January 22, 1980. In his report, Dr Dudiak cited three of his goals for the medical staff which had either been achieved during this past year or are now in progress. The first was to update and enhance our quality

> assurance program. Toward that goal, members of the medical staff attended an InterQual Conference in Chicago designed for quality assurance functions of the medical staff. Later, a faculty member from InterQual was invited to visit our hospital to conduct an on-site survey. As a result of these efforts, a centralized, more streamlined hospital-wide approach to quality assurance has now been begun with the establishment of a new staff quality assurance committee under Dr. Paul Simenstad.
>
> In closing, Dr. Dudiak expressed his pleasure and personal appreciation for the high standards of excellence and for the loyalty of the medical staff. He also expressed his thanks to hospital administration for their continuing effort to improve the quality of patient care.
>
> **Stephen Dudiak, M.D.,**
> Chief of Staff
> Gerald Derus, M.D.,
> Chief Elect

February 27 Dr. Lou Bernhardt, a cardiovascular surgeon, and President of the Dean Clinic Medical Staff was kind enough to meet with me after patient hours.

Lou, I am trying to help the St. Mary's Medical Staff Leadership understand that the problems during Agnes Woodbury's two hospitalizations were not my fault, but the facts of her care need to be studied and used to help ensure that similar problems do not occur in the future.

Ira, I don't know anything about bone healing.

Lou, you split sternums. You know about bone healing, and the facts of her care are clearly evident.

[**Note:** *I had open heart surgery almost 20 years ago, and I know about "split sternums" all too well. If you ever have a heart surgeon, tell you he or she does not know about bone healing run.*]

But Lou Bernhardt, and a couple of other highly qualified, and highly respected members of that hospital medical staff, when they were nice enough to meet with me privately, and hear my concern, they, collectively, and individually, could not bring themselves to admit that their two colleagues had demonstrated such bad judgement. I had been a near neighbor of one of the most qualified Internist in Madison, and a leader at the Dean Clinic, and my meeting with him after meeting with Lou went the same way. There are rare exceptions to this most usual response, and I will include that after completing Agnes' story, we are only about halfway through her saga.

My letter to the St. Mary's Executive Committee, as requested.

March 10, 1980

Stephen Dudiak, M.D.
Chief of Staff
St. Mary's Hospital

Dear Dr. Dudiak,

I wish to thank you and the Executive Committee for allowing this matter of treatment of Mrs. Agnes Woodbury from July 1, 1979, to November 2, 1979, to remain open.

My reasons for disagreeing with the treatment rendered to Mrs. Woodbury during this period are:

A. *A complete lack of radio-graphic documentation during the four-month period, and*
B. *No evidence of any positive treatment directed toward the cause(s) of the complications existing on November 2, 1979, and*
C. *No evidence of any consultations from a qualified source, and*
D. *The fact was that Mrs. Woodbury's condition on November 2, 1979, was, in my judgement, worse after four months of treatment than it was on July 1, 1979.*

The above reasons must be tempered by the fact that I have not had access to the documents and have not made a detailed study of all the documents related to this case. Nor do I consider myself to be the ultimate local authority in the treatment of facial trauma.

My reasons for reservations concerning the proceedings of the January 29, 1980, Surgery Patient Review Committee meeting are:

A. *My letter submitted to Walter Baranowski, M.D., Chairman of that committee was not requested, nor was it ever submitted or intended to be utilized as the basis for such a meeting. I was told by Dr. Baranowski on the night of December 12, 1979 (our only meeting) that he would follow my recommendation of having this matter reviewed outside of the local professional community, and*

B. *I was never informed that my letter would be used as a basis for that meeting, and I was never invited to attend or requested to appear. I had no knowledge of the use of my letter until I was allowed to read the minutes of that meeting on Thursday, February 7, 1980, in the office of S.P. Vinograd, M.D., Medical Director, and*

C. *I was surprised to see on reading the minutes of that meeting, that while my letter was used as the basis for the meeting, no copy of that letter is attached to the minutes as an opart of the record, and*

D. *It was evident from the minutes that even thought I had delivered to Dr. Baranowski, upon his request in December 1979, four copies of my x-ray taken of Mrs. Woodbury on November 2, 1979, and the basis for all my concerns in this matter, no reference was made in the minutes to this important document, and*

E. *It is evident on reading the minutes of January 29, 1980, that the content of the meeting was incomplete. Only the hospital documents covering the St. Mary's admissions of July 1 and July 30, 1979, were discussed. My concerns involve the period July 1 to November 2, 1979, and can only be reviewed adequately by including all hospital and Dean Clinic charts, x-rays, etc.*

Because of the above I find the last statements contained in the letter of January 31, 1980, by Dr. Baranowski and that February 6, 1980, by Dr. Vinograd to be to be totally unacceptable.

Should the Executive Committee decide to reconvene the Surgery Patient Review Committee on this matter, and should the major change be my appearance, I feel that a great responsibility would be placed upon me in my obligations to my patient and my obligations to the hospital. While it should not be necessary in the normal functions of the established peer review procedures, I feel that I will be placed in an isolated, accuser position.

Therefore, I feel that certain ground rules must be considered and accepted.

A. *After the convening of the committee by the chairman, the meeting proper will be directed by myself, and*

B. *All parties present on January 29, 1980, will attend and complete co-operation by all presents will be assured, and*

C. *All hospital and clinic records and x-rays will be available to me one week prior to the meeting and all aspects of their contents may be used, and*

D. To ensure accurate and complete minutes of the proceedings and ensure the protection of all participants, the events of the meeting will be recorded by a legal stenographer hired by me and paid for by the hospital or a tape recorder controlled by me.

It has been brought to my attention by two different sources that James H. Brandenburg, M.D., Chief of Otolaryngology at the University of Wisconsin and Gordon Davenport, M.D. Chief of Surgery at Madison General Hospital and John E. Hamacher, M.D., both practicing plastic surgeons at St. May's Hospital with privileges in the treatment of facial trauma have in some way reviewed some aspects of Mrs. Woodbury's treatment. Perhaps they should be requested to attend.

While the Bylaws, Rules and Regulations of St. Mary's Hospital is replete with phrases such as, "a high level of performance of Medical Staff members", "continuous review and evaluation of the clinical hospital activities of the Medical Staff", and "specific consideration shall be given to each member with respect to his professional competency and clinical judgment in the treatment of his patients, his ethics and conduct, —". I feel that the established peer review procedures in the case of Mrs. Woodbury and, contrary to the opinion of Dr. Vinograd, have failed in the above matter.

I request that this letter and all correspondence mentioned in this letter be made a permanent part of the record concerning this matter.

I also request that the Executive Committee decide not to reconvene the Surgery Patient Review Committee within the framework of my guidelines that I be notified in writing as to that decision and the reasons used to reach that decision.

Should the course of event proceed in that direction, I will assume that my next level of appeal is to the Board of Directors of St. Mary's Hospital. I would appreciate guidelines on making such an appeal.

I deeply regret for all parties concerned that this matter has taken so long to be resolved. Perhaps these events will provide an improved mechanism for the established peer review procedures in future considerations.

I will attend your March 17, 1980, meeting.

Sincerely,
Ira E. Williams, D.D.S.

March 17, St. Mary's Executive Committee meeting, and it was also St. Patrick's Day, and my wife and I had been invited to a St. Pat's party. I told my wife that I would join her as soon as I could.

Picture a long room, with a long conference table, and seated, all looking at me were 16 doctors, all chiefs of their medical specialties, and two members of the hospital administration, and a place for me wedged in on a far corner, and far away from the door. I thought, "I now know how General Custer must have felt looking at all of those Indians coming at him."

I have a copy of the 21 legal pages transcript of my portion of that meeting, but my copy is dated 3/30/83. I only have a copy of that transcript because Agnes and her husband decided to initiate a medical malpractice lawsuit against Dr. Tom and Dr. Tim, and naturally I became their expert witness, but more on that aspect of Agnes' story when it will become relevant.

Also, what that document does not mention is that I was chosen to be the last item on that meeting's agenda, and therefore forced to sit silently, and uncomfortably as they proceeded through the regular business of their monthly Executive Committee meeting. My anticipated St. Pat's Day fun would have to wait.

Unlike previous documents, and letters that I have recorded in full, I will not transcribe the entire 21 legal pages text because so much of the discussions were superfluous to what should have been the true goal of any discussion regarding Agnes' 4 months, 2 hospitalizations, and 2 trips to the operating room.

Dr. Gerald Derus, Chief Elect of the Executive Committee chaired the meeting, and after introducing each member seated at the table to me, he said.

So, Dr. Williams, I think we will let you lead off and then we will entertain questions and hope that this item on the agenda will not take more than 30 minutes, although I will not restrict it if the discussion seems germane.

I didn't realize at the time that I would have an opening statement, but there are several points that I would like to get across to you and I am glad that I do. I am here at the pleasure of the executive committee as a member of your staff, and I think there are several things that we should cover so that you will know where I am coming from and why this has become so involved. Some of you know and some of you may not know that several years ago there was a "oral surgery problem in this hospital". That doesn't involve this. The point that I am most concerned about is the period from July 1, 1979, to November 2, 1979, regarding the treatment of Agnes Woodbury.

This is not a plot or anything I have produced; in fact, I am sorry it has come down to the fact that I should be here. One of the most unfortunate things that we have come down to with this problem is that your peer review system has been placed completely on my shoulders because of the events of the last few months. This is most unfortunate. But, when I view what my understanding is of the treatment given to Mrs. Woodbury during those four months, I feel I have only three options. I could turn my back after turning it over to Dr. Vinograd and forget it. I can do what I am doing now and have in the past or I can recommend that she seek regress in another area. If I were vindictive over the history of this hospital, I would have done the latter.

In my mind, we are talking about a very grave problem that involves the Dean Clinic, the hospital, and the men that dealt with the treatment here. As you review these materials, I want you to know that her care was turned over to me completely voluntarily, I had no idea when it was turned over to me that it would have involved anything like this. It wasn't planned. I am on your staff, I am now her primary care physician for this problem, I feel a distinct moral and ethical obligation to this lady and any future patients that might be treated here in this area. I can't walk away from her.

What I am doing is the only thing I feel I can do. I don't feel I am the D.A. of trauma care in the city, there is not a man here who doesn't have complications who need consults including myself. I need a lot of help. Plus, the fact; I have an extremely happy home and good practice and I don't need all of this hassle I have had for the last five months, four and a half months, but I can't walk away from this. The last thing I want to say is when you review this problem, you must understand that in my judgment these men were treating this lady with the best they could. They were giving her their best shot. There was no one looking over their shoulder and for this four-month period, you have to assume they were treating her the way they would treat anyone else. This concerns me greatly.

Dr. Derus: Thank you Ira. I think that, would you want to make any comments before we ask questions about the document dated January 29, 1980, that is the special meeting of the surgical patient review.

My comments: I have read the document twice in Dr. Vinograd's office, I haven't studied it, I haven't committed it to memory, but it is my opinion that the 16-man surgery patient review committee failed this hospital terribly in this matter and I feel because of that now, I feel that the peer review system has failed you because it is now on one person's shoulders and this isn't the way it should work. I am left with no other choice but to be the smoking gun here and I think it is unfortunate for anyone. So, as you review this, I hope you consider your entire peer review mechanism and how you expect it to work.

Beginning on page 5 and ending on page 10 is a lot of discussion about what should have been an irrelevant issue. Dr. Roggensack, Chief of Radiology at the hospital took great exception to the fact that I had said that the flat plate x-rays of Agnes' lower jaw taken on July 30, 1979, at the Dean Clinic were inadequate, and the Dean Clinic radiologist, a member of the Surgery Patient Review Committee had said his x-rays were so adequate, and a plastic surgery member of that committee supported that view.

I will attempt to clarify the x-ray issue here, once and for all, I hope. I was the person who strongly urged the then St. Mary's Hospital Chief of Radiology, and I don't remember his name, to add a Panorex x-ray machine to their department shortly after our surgery group had obtained one, and he (they) did.

Agnes was transferred from St. Clair Hospital in Baraboo, WI to St. Mary's on July 1, 11979, and both chest x-rays and a Panorex x-ray were taken upon her admission, and that Panorex x-ray demonstrated her mandibular fracture in great detail. Agnes would go on to be hospitalized at St. Mary's twice, and be taken to the operating room twice, and be diagnosed with a post-op infection during each hospitalization, and no post-op Panorex x-ray was ever taken. The Panorex x-ray taken at my office on November 2, 1979, was the first, and only post-op Panorex x-ray taken during the entire four months of treatment rendered by two board-certified surgeons. And two radiologists had their nose out of joint because I considered the flat plate x-rays taken at Dean Clinic on July 30, 1979, were inadequate, and compared to the Panorex x-rays they were. Yet all that time and talk was wasted on an insignificant matter.

Dr. Rudy, an orthopedic surgeon: What is the status of this woman now? (Page 12)

I saw her Saturday. She has a fair piece of interior boarder of the bone out, we do have clinical healing, she has some scar tissue in the area that is tender. Her mandible was reduced out of the occlusion she had before the accident, but it is something that dentally they think they can work with. She will never be the same as far as—she is a tough patient to work with. She is just scared. She has been through a lot. This lady went through almost six months of continuously draining jaw, and she had a non-union for all that time. We have clinical healing now; she has been off antibiotics since the middle of December and the next procedure that I plan now is in May to smooth the alveolus where it was set off a little bit so that she can have a dental partial way to rehabilitate herself.

The next three pages consisted of a very disjointed discussion regarding the use, non-use, and/or misuse of antibiotics, both by her Dean Clinic surgeons, and me, while there was no mention of the offending "tooth-in-the-line-of - fracture, the source of her consistent infection for the entire 4-month period of their treatment.

On page 15 there was some discussion regarding my comment that her surgeons had never sought consultation from a qualified source during the far-from-normal period of treatment. Her doctors had suggested that she see her dentist, but he did not treat mandibular fractures, and therefore, was not a qualified consultant.

Page 16 I was asked to comment, and was given an opportunity to briefly describe, step-by-step, her two hospitalizations, and related events leading up to my first seeing her on November 2.

Page 17 Dr. Rudy: Going over these records, when she was seen infrequently, do you think she was in a lot of pain in those four months? What causes you to describe this woman as being a bundle of nerves now, do you think it is due to her discomfort because she obviously didn't come back frequently? The only time she would come back was when she did have trauma, she was treated for that. During the four months do you think she was that uncomfortable?

She and her husband both commented to me that when she was in fixation, they had assumed that the fixation should be firm and hers was loose. She had had—I have not tried to talk too deeply with her, of course I have attempted to have no influence on what action she might do. I have tried to guard what I say to them at all times. I haven't tried to get too deep into that period for a purpose. My feeling was that my concern should be handled within the medical organization. So, I haven't gone too deeply into that period other than occasionally asking her a question here or there and she has been terribly uncomfortable from what I can gather.

I was then asked why I had delayed her admission into the hospital, and I explained that I had first seen her on Friday, the 2nd, late in the day. Had her return on the next Monday to remove the tooth in the line of fracture, and restart her on antibiotics, and then arrange an OR, and day for her admission into Methodist Hospital.

The transcript continues for several more pages, but the focus of the questions was on me, and not on what should have been the primary focus of the entire meeting; how two board-certified surgeons on their hospital's medical staff had so mistreated a simple, mandibular fracture for four months, and still left her worst off than the first day Dr. Tom saw her.

Also, so very important is that I was invited to meet with the Executive Committee, but I had not been given a copy of the Special Patient Review Committee report, but only allowed to read it in Dr. Vinograd's office, and no access to Dr. Tom's and Dr. Tim's Dean Clinic records, and all other clinic documents. So, I was the target of their "review", and not what really happened to Agnes in their hospital. Furthermore, none of Agnes' hospital or Dean Clinic records were available in the room for the committee members to see exactly what was being discussed. Was the process fair? No., Should I have expected it to be fair? No. But, they were in control so far.

This ill-conceived, so-called attempt to examine, and hopefully judge the quality of care rendered Agnes in their hospital, and clinic for a total of four months by the highest level of medical expertise ended as a sham, a perversion of what medical peer review should be about.

This meeting also ended any further, formal exchange between St. Mary's Leadership, and myself. All future communications took place by mail, but such communications did take place.

Medical Peer Review Ends

After two months, I could only assume that the St. Mary's Medical Staff Executive Committee had concluded that their March 17 meeting had been sufficient to finally put the matter of Agnes' quality of care provided by both her two hospitalizations, and her care at the Dean Clinic had been rendered in an acceptable manner, and it was time to move on to other considerations.

But the matter of the quality of Agnes' care was not a closed matter as far as I was concerned. Someway, I had come to understand that such a process as seeking peer review judgment could not be considered complete unless that process "touched all the bases". The Administrator of the hospital must be required to also render a judgment.

Also, like every other community, the Madison Medical Community included 3 private hospitals, the University of Wisconsin Hospital, and the VA hospital. And gossip typically made the rounds. Thus, it came to my attention that comments were coming out of the Dean Clinic that there was another oral surgeon in Madison who was more inclined to agree with the findings of the Surgery Patient Review Committee's conclusion that "the differences were one of judgment and not of inadequacy".

There was another group of 3 oral surgeons in Madison at that time, and while there was no hostility between the two groups, there was also no real comradeship between us. But I had heard that one of the oral surgeons in that other group had met with the Dean Clinic Chief of Staff and seemed to have been convinced that I was causing a problem where there was no real problem. Upon hearing this, I sent a copy of Agnes' November 2, 1979, Panorex x-ray taken in our office, and a short note to that oral surgeon, and received the following reply.

May 20, 1980

Ira,

Returning your x-ray. I certainly agree that as the course of events progressed that it was a serious mistake to not remove the tooth and provide better fixation/stabilization.

I plan to call Lou Bernhardt to make sure he understands my opinion as "another oral surgeon".

Thanks,
Jim

So, Dr. Lou, the cardiovascular surgeon who told me he didn't know anything about bone healing, even though he split sternums, had been looking for someone, anyone, qualified to speak about mandibular fractures who might be persuaded to support the findings of the Surgery Patient Review Committee. During this same time the following took place.

May 10, 1980

Stephen Dudiak, M.D.
Chief of Staff
St. Mary's Hospital

Dear Dr. Dudiak,

This letter is in regard to our telephone conversation of Friday, May 9, 1980.

I request and do strongly urge that I be permitted to attend the Executive Committee meeting of Monday, May 19, 1980.

I will assume and anticipate that I will take <u>no</u> part in the meeting except to observe. In fact, I will <u>not</u> participate unless a majority of the Executive Committee should for any reason request my participation.

> *Since there were persons present other than Executive Committee members at my meeting of March 17, 1980, and since it has <u>so</u> long to address my concerns regarding the care rendered Mrs. Woodbury, I do feel I have a right to attend as a non-participating observer.*
>
> *Sincerely,*
>
> **Ira E. Williams, D.D.S.**

Surprise, surprise! I was not invited to attend their May meeting, or any other meeting they may have had, and there may have been a big reason for them to distance themselves from me.

At that time, I was a member of a group of 5 oral surgeons, and none of my partners would have ever done what I had been doing, and none of them would have agreed with my efforts if asked. But one of my partners said to me that the Dean Clinic was considering suing our group because of my efforts in behalf of Agnes. I believed that there was no way the Dean Clinic would ever want this matter to become public, but my partners wanted something more tangible done, thus the following.

Minutes of June 11, 1980, Special Meeting

Discussion was had with respect to the treatment of Dr. Williams' patient, Mrs. Woodbury, by ENTs at the Dean Clinic, and Dr. Williams' reports regarding that care to the appropriate committee at St. Mary's Hospital.

It was agreed that Dr. Williams was acting in his own personal capacity, and not as an employee, officer, director, or shareholder of Oral Surgery, S.C., in bringing the treatment of Mrs. Woodbury to the attention of St. Mary's, and Oral Surgery, S.C., specifically disclaims any participation in this regard.

Oral Surgery, S.C., determined not to become involved or participate in any future attempts with respect to reporting the treatment or to authorize Dr. Williams to act on its behalf. It was agreed that all future actions of Dr. Williams in this regard would be in his own personal capacity.

Dated this 11th day of June 1980.

Signed by myself and my 4 partners.

Dean Clinic never sued, and Dean Clinic would have never sued, but this episode takes one behind the curtain of the real medical profession, and this is not an aberration.

It was obvious that no one at St. Mary's or Dean Clinic ever understood, or probably never wished to understand, my true motives for all my actions, even though some of them may have unintentionally been misguided. I sincerely wanted to help them begin to provide far better care for facial trauma patients. By the late 1970s I had been doing major jaw surgery for the correction of jaw deformities, and I had performed more intra-oral bone grafts than any other surgeon in Wisconsin. Yet the Plastic and ENT surgeons continued to dominate ER rooms and continued to harm too many patients with facial trauma injuries.

Therefore, when Dr. Dudiak, in his Annual Report, mentioned that Dr. Paul Simenstad would Chair the new Quality Assurance Committee I contacted Paul, and offered to help him, if interested, in conducting a retroactive review of mandibular fractures, and he agreed.

June 25, 1980, I have a copy of the letter I sent to Paul providing a Sample Criteria for Short-Stay Hospital Review. I won't bother to include that letter here, but it can be made available, if necessary.

Likewise, I have a copy of a two-page letter from Paul on Dean Clinic letterhead, dated July 3, 1980, headed, Dear Ira, and thanking me for my help in his conducting his review. But, the animosity by the Plastic and ENT surgeons toward oral surgeons, and their Turf War was too great to ever overcome; The contents of his letter are also available, if necessary. But, back to medical peer review at St. Mary's Hospital. We are approaching the end of that highly fractured process seeking to judge the care of a simple, fractured mandible on a middle-aged woman.

> July 2, 1980
>
> **Dr. Stephen Dudiak**
> Chief of Staff
> St. Mary's Hospital
>
> Dear Dr. Dudiak,
>
> I regret that the matter regarding Mrs. Agnes Woodbury's treatment has persisted so long.
>
> My interest can be summed up in, "Does the treatment rendered Mrs. Woodbury at St. Mary's Hospital during July and August 1979 meet the standard of care of St. Mary's Hospital for patients treated for mandibular fractures?"
>
> I would appreciate your consideration of the above at the July Executive Committee meeting.
>
> I look forward to hearing from you.
>
> Sincerely,
> **Ira E. Williams, D.D.S.**

(This letter was hand delivered to the Medical Staff Secretary. She said she would see that Dr. Dudiak received it.)

Surprise, surprise! No response. I was dead to them, or probably, they wished that I was dead, but I didn't go away.

> August 4, 1980
>
> **Governing Board**
> St. Mary's Hospital
> St. Louis, MO 63117
>
> Dear Sisters,
>
> I am writing to you regarding Mrs. Agnes Woodbury of Baraboo, Wisconsin.
>
> Mrs. Woodbury was a patient at St. Mary's Hospital, Madison, Wisconsin, with admissions on July 1, 1979, and July 30, 1979.

Mrs. Woodbury's care was transferred to me voluntarily on November 2, 1979, by her attending physician who had treated her during her two previous admissions.

In early December 1979, I contacted the St. Mary's Medical Director concerning the great reservations I had regarding the care rendered Mrs. Woodbury from July 1, 1979, to November 2, 1979.

To date there has been;

Special meeting of the Surgery Patient Review Committee, January 29, 1980.

Special Ad Hoc Committee of the Surgical Patient Review Committee, March 14, 1980.

St. Mary's Hospital Executive Committee meeting of March 17, 1980.

Quality Assurance Committee meeting of June 24, 1980.

The minutes of the above meetings demonstrate an inadequate specific review of the unprofessional aspects of Mrs. Woodbury's treatment during the specified period.

The minutes of the meeting of 1-29-80 and 3-14-80 exhibit definite examples of misrepresentation of fact.

The Executive Committee has accepted the Quality Assurance Committee meeting of 6-24-80 as the final review of these matters.

As a member (Courtesy) in good standing of the Medical Staff of St. Mary's Hospital, I request that the Governing Board completely review all events concerning the treatment of Mrs. Woodbury at St. Mary's and the reviews into her treatment, a period of July 1, 1979, to the present.

I also request that I be permitted to actively participate in the Governing Board's review.

I would appreciate personal contact with Sister Marie Michel Crooks, if possible.

Sincerely,
Ira E. Williams, D.D.S.

(This letter was sent by certified mail on August 5, 1980, and the return card was dated August 7, 1980

Surprise, surprise! No response.

August 24, Sunday evening, I obtained the phone number, and called the Mother House.)

> "Hello,
>
> Sister, I am Dr. Ira Williams in Madison, Wisconsin.
>
> Sister Rebecca will be in touch with you."
>
> (End of call)

August 27, 1980

Ira E. Williams, D.D.S.
416 W. Mifflin Street
Madison, WI 53703

Dear Dr. Williams,

The Governing Board of Saint Mary's Hospital Medical Center has received your letter to them dated August 4, 1980. I am responding to your letter on their direction.

The content of your letter was reviewed at a regular Board meeting as well as with St. Mary's Hospital Medical Center personal.

The Board maintains ongoing awareness of the Quality Assurance program at Saint Mary's Hospital Medical Center. The Board has been made aware of the proceedings and evaluations which have taken place up to this point.

It sems quite clear that the matters you raised have been thoroughly reviewed at the appropriate levels within the Medical Staff and administrative structure at St. Mary's Hospital Medical Center. The points that you have raised have received full and adequate review and evaluation. That peer review and analysis has been jointly completed.

> *The Board regards the action of the Joint Quality Assurance Committee as final and therefore will not accept your request to re-open this matter.*
>
> *Sincerely,*
> **Sister Rebecca Wright, S.S.M.**
> *Chief Executive Officer*

There, I finally had it! Every level of the St. Mary's Hospital Medical Center had stated in writing that Agnes' 4 month of treatment at their hospital was accepted to have met their standard of care for mandibular fractures. Good luck people in Madison, Wisconsin who might, at some time in the future, suffer a mandibular fracture, and be admitted to St. Mary's Hospital. Well, wait and see what happened only months after Sister Rebecca wrote her letter. It is unbelievable, but Agnes' story is far from over. As the song goes, "We've only just begun."

I had been saying nothing to Agnes and her husband about my on-going efforts in the pursuit of medical peer review, but I had hoped I might participate in a far more professional form of peer review. Obviously, that never happened, and, obviously, professional peer review at St. Mary's where the interests of the patient should receive equal consideration would also never take place.

St. Mary's NEWSLETTER, October issue informed that the Joint Commission was scheduled to survey St. Mary's Hospital in November, and individual staff and employee members could request an opportunity to be interviewed by the Survey Team Leader upon request. I thought, one more step in seeking professional peer review for Agnes.

> *October 27, 1980*
>
> **Mr. John Milton**
> *Vice President*
> *Hospital Accreditation*
> *Joint Commission on Accreditation of Hospitals*

> Dear Mr. Milton,
>
> It is my understanding that St. Mary's Hospital, Madison, Wisconsin will undergo its Biannual JCAH review during the last week of November 1980.
>
> As a courtesy member (dental) of St. Mary's Surgery Department I wish to request an individual meeting with the physician in charge of that review.
>
> I would appreciate hearing from you.
>
> Sincerely,
>
> **Ira E. Williams, D.D.S.**

Our office secretary took the following note on 10-30-80.

Dr. Williams, please call Helen Garvey from the Joint Commission regarding your letter. 1-312-642-6061, ext. 261, Deb.

And I called his office and spoke with Helen Garvey.

> November 4, 1980
>
> **Ira E. Williams, D.D.S.**
> Oral Surgery, S.C.
> 416 W. Mifflin Street
> Madison, Wisconsin 53703
>
> Dear Doctor Williams,
>
> A Public Information Interview has been scheduled for you at St. Mary's Hospital, Madison, Wisconsin. The date of the survey is November 21, 24, and 25, 1980.
>
> Enclosed you will find a copy of the Joint Commission's policy and procedures for conducting such interviews. Please note that it is the responsibility of the facility to notify the interviewees of the exact time, place, and date of the interview. Your request will be forwarded to the administrator for his implementation. Our surveyors will also be informed.

Sincerely,
Helen T. Garvey

November 17, 1980

JCAH Representative
St. Mary's Hospital
Madison, WI 53715

Dear Doctor,

As a courtesy member (dental) of the St. Mary's Surgery Department I have requested an individual interview during the biannual Joint Commission for the Accreditation of Hospitals review.

The subject of my concern is Mrs. Agnes Woodbury of Baraboo, Wisconsin. Mrs. Woodbury's care was transferred to me voluntarily on November 2, 1979. My concerns involve:

I. The care rendered Mrs. Woodbury from July 1, 1979, to November 2, 1979. This period includes two hospitalizations at St. Mary's for treatment of the same problem and,

II. The "peer review" rendered her care at my request during the period of December 3, 1979, to August 27, 1980.

My reasons for disagreeing with the treatment rendered Mrs. Woodbury during this period are:

A. A complete lack of adequate post-operative radiographic documentation during the four-month period, and
B. No evidence of any positive treatment directed toward the cause(s) of the complications existing on November 2, 1979, and
C. No evidence of any consultations from a qualified source, and
D. No evidence of proper isolation and care on either admission despite evidence and treatment of persistent infection, and
E. Oral evidence from the patient that she was not seen by a primary care physician in the hospital immediately after the second surgery (August 7, 1979) and was discharged by phone on August 10, 1979, and
F. The fact that Mrs. Woodbury's condition on November 2, 1979, was, in my judgment, worse after four months of treatment than it was on July 1, 1979.

> *Should you or the JCAH require additional information, please contact me.*
>
> *Sincerely,*
> **Ira E. Williams, D.D.S.**

I repeat, because I believe it bears repeating, I had told Agnes, and her husband *nothing* about any of my "peer review" activities throughout our many meetings through the course of my treatment for her injury because I truly believed the two activities, my treatment of her, and my professional responsibility to the St. Mary's Hospital Medica Staff and Administration should be kept separate. But since St. Mary's Hospital had documented satisfaction with the care, she had received during the course of four months, "they", not I, had closed the book on the peer review of the care rendered Mrs. Agnes Woodbury at their hospital.

I had been scheduled to meet with the JCAH physician in charge of the survey team on November 25, 1980. I called Agnes and asked if I could come to Baraboo, and meet she and her husband, and she said yes. I met with them on November 24. Agnes, I am scheduled to meet with the doctor in charge of the Joint Commission survey team at St. Mary's Hospital tomorrow afternoon. Would you like to join me at that meeting?

Yes, Doctor Williams. My husband and I have been considering getting an attorney to consider a lawsuit against St. Mary's Hospital and both Dr. Tom and Dr. Tim. So, yes, I would like to see how the Joint Commission might react to what I went through for all those many months.

I still remember Agnes and I walking up the steps to enter the front door of St. Mary's Hospital, and walking into the cafeteria, and sitting down at a small table with Dr. Vinograd, the St. Mary's Hospital Medical Director and the Joint Commission doctor seated across from us. Dr. Vinograd had a slight smile on his face as it he was thoroughly enjoying this miniature theater.

Agnes was understandably nervous, and I would have preferred to be any place else, but I felt this was one more vital step in the process I had initiated 12 months earlier. I gave the JCAH doctor my letter, and Agnes attempted to describe the months of distress, and discomfort she had been forced to endure for so long, and the two doctors just sat there as though they were enjoying not only the entire process, but also our obvious discomfort. Agnes and I were there about 20 minutes, and when we left, I went away with a profound feeling of disgust. I felt we had been treated like insignificant pests, but we had taken one more step in the process to demonstrate medical peer review in its reality.

Surprise, surprise! Again, no response from the JCAH, or St. Mary's Hospital, St. Mary's NEWSLETTER, February 1981. Joint Commission had given St. Mary's Hospital a statement that their hospital was in full compliance with all Joint Commission standards, and the new Chief of Staff, Dr. Gerald Derus could not have been more proud.

> *February 18, 1981*
> **Gerald Derus, M.D.**
> *Chief of Staff*
> *St. Mary's Hospital*
>
> *Dear Dr. Derus,*
>
> *Mrs. Agnes Woodbury, Baraboo, Wisconsin, and I attended a Public Information Interview with the Joint Commission during its November survey of St. Mary's Hospital.*
>
> *It is fully understood by Mrs. Woodbury and myself that while all information obtained by the Joint Commission during the survey process is confidential between the JCAH and the hospital, we also understand that the hospital can make available the JCAH report to persons with sufficient need to know.*
>
> *Mrs. Woodbury and I would appreciate my access to only that portion of the JCAH report dealing with the Public Information Interview we participated in.*
>
> *Sincerely,*
> **Ira E. Williams, D.D.S.**

> March 4, 1981
>
> **I.E. Williams, D.D.S.**
> 416 W. Mifflin Street
> Madison, WI 53703
>
>
> Dear Dr. Williams,
>
> St. Mary's Hospital Medical Center received written communication from the Joint Commission on Accreditation of Hospitals on February 24, 1981. The full two-year accreditation was granted.
>
> In reviewing the entire document, there was no mention made of the public information interview in which you and Mrs. Woodbury participated. I appreciate your concern of issues that have been brought to our attention in regard to quality care patient review. I shall do everything in my power to continue the tradition here at St. Mary's in an effort to put the patient first at all times.
>
>
> Sincerely,
> **G.J. Derus, M.D.**

Agnes and her husband would sue the doctors, and St. Mary's Hospital, but not, unfortunately in a normal, civil court proceedings.

Medical and dental practitioners were happily practicing their trade, and minding their business when the Professions were blindsided by a tsunami in the mid-1970s. The first wave of the Medical Malpractice Crisis hit without warning. Some malpractice insurers went out of business, and the ones that survived began to write their malpractice coverage in two different forms, and at much higher prices.

Tsunami is an accurate way to view the Medical Malpractice Crisis of the 70s because, like a tsunami, the second wave of that crisis would pass through the Professions in the early 80s, and other, smaller waves would follow. In fact, in my opinion, that Medical Malpractice Crisis has never ceased to exist, and the fundamental problems of medical malpractice litigation are still as bad now as it has always been, but that is the subject for another book.

Wisconsin Legislature, true to form, never let a crisis go unnoticed, and they created a new form of medical malpractice review; Medical Malpractice Panels, and their structure may be hard to believe.

If the Plaintiff's Complaint was for $10,000 or less, the panel would consist of one attorney, acting as Chief Counsel, one physician member, and one lay person member.

If the Plaintiff's Complaint was for more than $10,000, the panel would consist of one attorney, acting as Chief Counsel, two physician members, and two lay person members.

Agnes and her husband naturally sued for more than $10,000, and therefore became the victims of the expanded form of Medical Malpractice Panels.

I would be Agnes' only Plaintiff's Expert Witness. But doctors always find it easy to obtain highly qualified expert witnesses to appear on their behalf.

Doctors Donovan, and St. Mary's Expert Witness list, including themselves:

James Brandenburg, M.D.,
Chairman, ENT Department,
Un Wisconsin Hospital

David Dibbell, M.E.,
Chairman, Plastic Surgery Department,
Un Wisconsin Hospital.

Jerry Schmitz, M.D.,
Chairman, ENT Department,
Medical College of Wisconsin, Milwaukee.

Louis Gallio, M.D.,
Chairman of ENT Department,
University of California at Davis, CA.

> **George Roggensack, M.D.**
> Radiologist,
> St. Mary's Hospital

Each of these medical experts were ready to testify, under oath, that the care rendered to Agnes Woodbury at St. Mary's Hospital, and Dean Clinic between July 1 and November 2, 1979, met a reasonable, and acceptable standard of care, and that standard of care had been validated by every level of medical and administrative leadership at that hospital. Welcome to the real world of medical malpractice litigation.

The Panel was convened for three days, June 15-17, 1983, and three years after her treatment. The good news is that both surgeons and the hospital were found guilty of negligence.

The bad news is that Panel awarded Agnes and her husband a negligible amount of money for all her suffering, and despair.

I would participate in another Wisconsin Medical Malpractice Panel disgrace, again as the second surgeon, and only Plaintiff's expert witness, a few years later that would closely resemble Agnes' Panel in scope and result. It is my understanding that the Wisconsin Legislature eliminated those Panels later in the 1980s.

But I want to go back to the root cause of the professional, or rather unprofessional conflict between the medical head and neck surgeons in Madison, and the oral surgeons.

Now that Agnes' peer review process has come to an end, I feel it is time to offer some perspective review of what was mentioned earlier in Agnes' story, and that is the turf war, or hostility shown by both ENT and plastic surgeons toward oral surgeons, or "those dentist".

When I joined the Oral Surgery, S.C. group in 1966 the norm was that oral surgeons provided dental surgery with general anesthesia when requested, and the plastic and ENT surgeons in the city made sure the dental surgeons were never called to treat patients with facia trauma in the hospital ERs. But, with the advent of more advanced surgical procedures by oral surgeons, my inclusion in the city, and my request for hospital medical staff privileges initiated clear signs of unprofessional efforts to severely limit oral surgeons' privileges to new arrivals such as myself.

I was able to gain courtesy medical staff privileges at each of the three hospitals in Madison, but a message had been sent during those separate processes that I was expected to emulate my partners in limiting my surgical efforts to our clinic practice. All of that would begin to change after 1970 when I became board-certified, and particularly after my very successful one-week mini-residency.

1971 I began to perform surgical correction of jaw deformities, all at Methodist Hospital at first because that hospital had created a Dental Department and put the Chairman of that Department on the Medical Staff Executive Committee.

1972 St. Mary's Hospital Medical Staff, and the Dean Clinic ENT surgeons initiated the opening shot that would lead to a brief, but continuous face-off between the medical surgeons and the oral surgeons of the city by creating an AD HOS COMMITTEE, and a statement of surgery limitations.

Naturally, I took exception to this unilateral power grab, and thus, I became the point-man in letting the St. Mary's Medical Staff Chief of Staff know that the contents of that document were unacceptable. I was invited to attend the next St. Mary's Executive Committed meeting.

When I walked into the room full of doctors seated around the conference table, with me was a friend, and one of the most aggressive trail attorneys in Madison. One might have thought that he and I had entered the room with no clothes on. But I got my point across. I was willing to discuss our differences, but I would not be dictated to.

The Chief of Staff stated that they had not anticipated an attorney would participate in our meeting and asked that Don please leave. Both Don and I thought that was agreeable since his presence had redirected any future discussions. I remained, and a rather muddled discussion was attempted. The essence was that more discussion would be necessary, and I agreed. In the meantime, the plastic and ENT surgeons at both Madison General Hospital, and St. Mary's Hospital had formed the AD HOC Committee, and the following document stated their perception of the privilege boundaries should be for oral surgeons in Madison, Wisconsin.

REPORT FROM AD HOC COMMITTEE

Privileges for Oral Surgeons within the Hospital Emergency Room Policy

1) They should be called on trauma patients only as a consultant and not as a primary physician.
2) They may consult on a trauma patient only after the primary physician has personally attended the patient.
3) They may not become the primary physician for any patients admitted to the hospital for trauma.

OPERATIVE SURGERY

1) The following, we feel, are within the scope of a dentist practicing oral surgery.
   - Closed reductions of mandible fractures.
   - Open reductions of fractures of the body of the mandible.
   - Closed reductions on the tooth-bearing portion of the maxilla, (LeForte I).
2) They should be allowed to perform:
   - Surgical removal and management of diseased teeth and ectopic denticians.
   - Preprosthetic surgery includes alveolectomies, alveoloplasties, vestibuloplastics, and phrenectomies.
   - Incision and drainage of abscesses.
   - Excision of benign tumors of the mouth and mandible.
3) The following, we feel, are beyond the scope of oral surgery:
   - Open reduction of the nose, maxilla, zygoma, orbital floor or orbital rim.
   - Temporomandibular joint surgery.
   - Salivary gland surgery.
   - Correction of facial clefts
   - Prognathism as a general rule. In exceptional cases when a man shows adequate formal training, he

should be given special consideration in certain types of prognathism.
4) They should not treat any patients for cancer whether this be a biopsy or definitive treatment. This precludes biopsy distortion of the original boundaries of the tumor prior to assigning the patient to the care of the man who will treat him.

These recommendations have been developed in keeping with the high standards of practice in the Madison area and are not intended to hinder any oral surgeon in the practice of dental oral surgery.

Signed: Tim J. Donovan, M.D.

So, the medical head & neck surgeons of Madison assumed that oral surgeons, due to their inferior degree, should be under the paternal guidance of their medical colleagues. Such thinking was totally unacceptable.

December 11, 1972

Mr. Donald S. Eisenberg
Attorney at Law
Re: Oral Surgery Privileges

Dear Mr. Eisenberg,

This will confirm our telephone conversation of the afternoon of Friday, December 8, wherein it was agreed that in lieu of your group meeting with the Executive Committee on Thursday, December 14, they would meet with the Plastic Surgery and the Ear, Nose and Throat Groups. It was understood that all members of each group would be present. I also intend to be present and assume that you will likewise be there. It is hopeful that there might be some meaningful discussions between the interested parties to the end that this controversy might be resolved in a professional manner.

Very truly yours,
Eugene O. Gehl

December 14 the "informal meeting" was held at St. Mary's Hospital. Attending were the two attorneys, Dr. Max Smith, St. Mary's Hospital Chief of Staff, and the following surgeons.

- 3 Plastic Surgeons from Madison General Hospital, and Dr. Gordon Davenport as Ad Hoc Chairman of their group.
- 3 ENT Surgeons from Madison General Hospital
- 3 ENT Surgeons from St. Mary's Hospital
- 5 Oral Surgery Surgeons, 4 from Oral Surgery SC, and a solo oral surgeon who came to Madison in 1968, and practiced alone, but not for long.
- One legal transcription reporter

I have in my possession the entire, bound 80-page copy of the proceedings of that evening, but I will spare readers with that record of a group of men trying to settle their differences when neither side wanted to give an inch. The unacknowledged factor during the entire evening's discussions was that I had introduced attorneys into the discussion, and those medical surgeons had no desire to be forced to conclude this problem in a court of law.

The result was that, yes, a formal agreement was adopted and signed by all parties in the coming days, but the plastic surgeons at Madison General Hospital, and ENT surgeons, particularly at St. Mary's Hospital passively ignored it.

In the coming years I would be performing surgeries that none of that group of medical surgeons could ever attempt, and I would have an opportunity to perform a few such surgeries at Madison General Hospital, but never at St. Mary's Hospital. But I did come close to possibly performing a surgical correction for the surgical correction of a prognathic mandible there.

1974 Bernard came to my office for a consultation. He had recently become a Seminarian student at the Catholic Seminary in Middleton, at the west end of Lake Mendota. He said his family lived in a rural area West of Madison, and he had no healthcare coverage from his family, or from the Seminary.

Bernard had a severe Class III, or prognathic mandibular over-bite, and it was obvious that this deformity had created a great psychological impact for him, and he wanted to know if I could help him.

Bernard, yes, I will perform your surgery at no charge, if you will promise to pray for me and my family while at the Seminary, and as a priest. (My wife and I, and our sons were practicing Catholics.) And I will call St. Mary's and see if they will provide the hospital coverage.

So, I called St. Mary's Hospital, and spoke with a person in the Administration Office, and recounted Bernard's plight, and said that I would perform the surgery at no cost, and could they provide the hospital services at no cost for this young Seminarian in such great need?

Absolutely not! We can't provide free hospitalizations. It is out of the question.

As a practicing Catholic that refusal was a bitter pill to swallow, but where could I turn. I went to see my friend Bill Johnson, Methodist Hospital Administrator.

Bill, I have this young Seminarian student who is in great need for corrective surgery, and I have offered to perform the surgery for no charge, but St. Mary's said they could not provide the hospitalization for no charge even to a Seminary student. Can you help us?

Yes Ira! And no problem. We will use Hill-Burton funds. The Hill-Burton Bill was passed by Congress several years ago for just such healthcare need, and we would be happy to cover his hospital costs.

Thus, Bernard got his surgery, and hospitalization at no cost, and I missed what would prove to be my only chance to perform major surgery at St. Mary's Hospital. After his surgery, and six-weeks of inter-maxillary fixation, and firm healing, I removed all his wires and arch bars, and he left my office without even a thank you. I never saw or heard from Bernard again. Several years later my family and I would go with a group of other families to the Seminary for Christmas-eve midnight mass, and there was no sight of Bernard. I can only hope his surgery helped him find a better life.

Yes, my activities, and the events depicted thus far took place 40 years ago, and yes, my activities, and those events laid the foundation for my becoming an author of 4 books on the HCDS, and a sufficient student of that "System" to claim I understand Why and How that system is and has always been greatly flawed.

But we currently find ourselves in the 3rd decade of the 21st century, and 40 years is a long time, so why is Agnes' story, and all that goes with that story, still relevant today? To connect the dots to what has taken place in the on-going efforts to improve the Quality of Care and Patient Safety within that system one must be introduced to the Quality of Care and Patient Safety army of experts.

Unbelievable

Dr. Tom, the younger brother, had seemed contrite, and genuinely moved by his and his brother's 4-month long travesty with Agnes, and I assumed he had recognized that the only difference between their treatment of Agnes' injury, and my successful treatment was that I had removed the tooth in the line of fracture prior to surgically correction her long-standing non-union. There had been NO magic, just remove the tooth that had been the source of all of her infection throughout those months, and her body was capable of doing the rest. But Dr. Tom had not recognized that simple difference between their treatment, and my treatment, and exactly two years after his negligent treatment of Agnes, he would proceed to demonstrate patient care stupidity beyond belief, and he would not be alone in doing so. Dr. Tom, his family dentist, and an infectious disease Dr. on the Medical Staff would collaborate in one of the most stupid examples of patient care, and in the process begin to destroy a young man's life, and never pay for it. IF this introduction seems too severe, trust me, it is not.

James, a 25-year-old truck driver happened to visit the same tavern on July 11, 1981, as his ex-wife, and her new other, and words were said, and violence erupted. James ended up at the St. Mary's Emergency Room at 2:30 a.m., and unfortunately for him, Dr. Tom was on call. James must have been hit square on the chin, and that blow resulted in him have a fracture just like

Agnes' fracture, but his lower jaw was fractured on both sides, and there was a tooth in the line of each fracture, and anyone reading this book knows that when Dr. Tom, a lower jaw fracture (even on one side), and with a tooth in the line of fracture, one should prepare for the worst, and that is just what happened to James.

Exactly two years, and ten days after Dr. Tom had admitted Agnes for a lower jaw fracture, he now admitted James with bilateral lower jaw fractures. Dr. Tom's INPATIENT ADMISSION RECORD shows that he had learned his lesson well because he admitted James with two Consulting Physicians who had agreed to share his patient-care responsibilities.

Dr. Giswold, a general dentist with no formal surgical training was apparently added to his dental expertise, and he would assist Dr. Tom in the operating room during the first surgery three days after admission.

Dr. Hetsko's name is familiar because he was a member of the Surgery Patient Review Committee that had met on January 29, 1980, and they had unanimously agreed that the differences between my care of Agnes, and Drs. Tom and Tim's care of Agnes were one of judgment and not of inadequacy. But there is far more about Dr. Hetsko; his specialty is *infectious disease*, and his inclusion as a Consulting Physician three days before the first surgical correction of James' injuries is an unbelievable, but prophetic judgement by Dr. Tom that his treatment of jaw fractures typically resulted in post-operative infections, and his prediction proved to be correct. James' treatment of his jaw fractures by a board- certified ENT surgeon, a general dentist, and an infectious disease specialist would prove to be a total disaster for their patient. And again, a second surgeon would have to provide corrective surgery for James' injuries, but not before James had been forced to endure unbelievable torture at the hands of three licensed practitioners as they demonstrated their incompetence.

There is a need to stop, and fully consider what took place on James' first day of admission to St. Mary's Hospital. Apparently, Dr. Tom anticipated that his, and his family dentist's treatment would, like Agnes' treatment, result in his patient becoming post-operatively infected, so he asked his fellow medical staff member, and infectious disease expert to sign the Inpatient Admission Record as a treating physician. I don't know which is the most unbelievable, that Dr. Tom would ask such a specialist to join him at the patient's admission, and prior to any treatment, or that such a specialist would accept such a request. I had previously referred to the two ENT brothers as Drs. Dumb and Dumber, but Dr. Hetsko's willing participation in James' admission prior to any treatment adds a new, and very telling addition to the previously established accepted standard of care for the treatment of lower jaw fractures to included post-operative infections as being anticipated at St. Mary's Hospital. Forty years later, and it is still difficult to imagine how three practicing caregivers could demonstrate stupid negligence of the highest degree, and for so long, while the entire St. Mary's Hospital Medical Staff remained silent.

James' first surgery would take place on July 14, 1981, and Dr. Tom would be assisted by Dr. Tim, and Dr. Giswold would provide the necessary dental expertise to see that his jaws were wired closed "in as near perfect occlusion as possible." Keep in mind that my treatment of Agnes' infected, non-union, involved surgery, and discharge from the Methodist Hospital in two days, and 6-weeks later, the arch bars and wires were removed along with the Bi-Phase pins, and her lower jaw was finally, after almost six months, healed. But I didn't have an infectious disease doctor helping me.

James' medical record Progress Notes contain numerous notes by Dr. Tom, Dr. Giswold, and Dr. Hetsko, and they document a series of events like those during Agnes' care, early signs of post-operative infection. But unlike in Agnes' care, Dr. Hetsko was there to supervise I.V. antibiotic treatment. Also, as in Agnes' care, James required a second trip to the OR on July 21, and again, Dr. Tom was assisted by Dr. Tim, and Dr. Giswold was there to provide dental expertise.

James' medical record Progress Notes would continue with numerous notes by Dr. Tom, while Dr. Hetsko was supervising his antibiotic meds for almost 3 more weeks, and until James said, enough is enough. As an employed truck driver, he had to get back to work.

James was told he must sign a document stating he was discharging himself out of the hospital *against medical advice* (AMA). That document was witnessed by Dr. Hetsko, and it would later be used as evidence that all of his previous treatment, and all of his future treatment for his lower jaw fractures could never be considered negligent care, even though all of the treatment he had received for the past 4 weeks, and all of the future treatment he would later receive at St. Mary's Hospital was, and would be negligent, and worthy of being considered criminally negligent, but never in a Wisconsin court. James signed that document on August 8, 1981, but that did not free him from further negligent care by those two doctors and one dentist.

Both Dr. Tom and Dr. Hetsko dictated separate Discharge Summaries describing in great detail all of James' past treatment, including both trips to the OR for surgeries that both proved to be incompetent, each report stated how James should have remained in the hospital for continuous antibiotic treatment, even though his lower jaw infections demanding far more definitive treatment that neither Dr. Tom or dental expert Dr. Giswold were capable of providing.

James returned to work, but with a continuously infected, and non-union fracture of his lower jaw for the remainder of August, and into early September. He was seen in consultation by my then partner at our downtown office, and again by me in that same office the next week. I was very careful in my comments to him and said nothing about my experience with Dr. Tom and Agnes, but I did tell him that he needed additional surgery, and that he must choose who he desired to be that next surgeon.

James was re-admitted to St. Mary's Hospital by Dr. Tom on September 21, and seen in consultation by my partner Dr. Joe, where he was diagnosed with a non-union of his lower jaw fracture. He was discharged the next day with the understanding that Dr. Joe would admit him to Methodist Hospital for additional surgery. Dr. Joe would provide similar surgical correction to James' lower jaw that I had used in correction Agnes' non-union two years previously.

Two years later James would obtain the services of an attorney and initiate a medical malpractice suit, and I would receive a complete copy of all the related records for his suit as his acting plaintiff's expert witness. But James, like that middle-aged lady in Columbus Ohio, would never receive his day in court because of that *against medical advice* document he was forced to sign.

Agnes, James, that lady in Columbus, Ohio, the Dean of Harvard Dental School's patient, and so many others are just a few examples of the Dark Side of the Healthcare Delivery System; the side of medicine that no one wants to talk about.

Agnes was the first, but not the last patient for whom I was to become the second surgeon tasked with the responsibility to surgically correct gross negligence caused by the first surgeon (all MDs), and each one at one of the other of the three private hospitals in Madison at that time. And the circumstances of those other two cases did not permit me an opportunity to try to initiate peer review within those hospital medical staffs.

The second case began the year before I first met Agnes, but my services as the second surgeon for that unfortunate individual did not begin until 1984, and that patient's malpractice litigation process would also be heard within that disgrace Wisconsin Special Medical Malpractice System. During my testimony during that trial, I described the original surgery as being "surgical mutilation". This case too, is a long story, and there is so much that needs to be said, and that could be learned from my experiences within the Madison Wisconsin Healthcare Delivery System for over two decades because I was able to participate inside the Dark Side of several hospital medical staffs, and see the truth as to why our current system is now, and has always been "broken" (a poor word for such a critical understanding, but it certainly conveys a stark understanding).

Yes, my activities, and the events depicted thus far took place 40 years ago, and yes, my activities, and those events laid the foundation for my becoming an author of 4 books on the HCDS, and a sufficient student of that "System" to claim I understand Why and How that system is and has always been greatly flawed.

But we currently find ourselves in the third decade of the 21st century, and 40 years is a long time, so why is Agnes' story, and all that goes with that story, still relevant today? The relevance of Agnes' story remain because of what Healthcare experts have been saying and doing, and not doing throughout those past decades. Agnes' story, and those other stories on the previous pages have been just snap shots taken from the enormous montage of how Your & Your Loved Ones Healthcare Delivery System functions and in too many cases fails to function effectively.

Since Congress created Medicare and Medicaid the Cost & Access aspect of healthcare, or how to pay for healthcare *after-the-fact* has been the overwhelming focus, while the healthcare rubber meets the road in the Healthcare Delivery System (HCDS), and at the doctor/patient interface. Yet the promises to improve the quality of care and patient safety, led by 5 Federal quality of care agencies since 1970 had been able to demonstrate NO evidence of patient safety improvement in over 3 decades prior to COVID. Clearly, something has been missing in all those efforts and promises, so it is time to closely examine some of those unkept promises.

None of my comments have been written in anger, but rather in candor. Now it's time to recognize what other Healthcare experts have been saying, and there can be no better person to guide us than the Father of Patient Safety, Dr. Lucian Leape (Leap), and his book, Making Healthcare Safe, The Story of the Patient Safety Movement.

Healthcare Stupidity

We of the electorate like to assume that a majority of those who volunteer to become elected decision-makers at local, state, or federal levels possess a better than average education and intelligence. But critical issues have the propensity to expose the negative characteristic of *selective stupidity*. Healthcare Delivery System (HCDS), and its inherent problems has provided a clear demonstration of that negative characteristic.

A vast army of Quality of Care and Patient Safety experts began to evolve when Congress replaced Doctors as the dominate force within hospitals due to the creation of Medicare and Medicaid in the mid-1960s, and how to pay for healthcare after-the-fact became more important than the quality of care those patients might be receiving. As those inherent problems within the HCDS rapidly became apparent, Congress began to create Federally funded Quality of Care and Patient Safety Agencies, with the first one joining the National Academies of Science, and Engineering, and first known as the Institute of Medicine (IOM) in 1970 but is currently known as the National Academy of Medicine, and while the name was changed, the incompetency has remained.

I have long had a great desire to write a book about that army of Quality of Care and Patient Safety experts, but I have been deterred by how to describe the vastness of that collection of entities, and the public's almost complete unawareness of its very existence, and thus, the prospects of there being any potential readers of such a book. That army of experts seem to exist in their own personal orbit within the Healthcare world like a stealth component, and their many contributions go unnoticed in the public's real world, and I will provide multiple examples to support this contention.

This army of experts really began to take its current form in the mid-1980s when the first, lengthy, and well-defined study of medical harm began in 1985 in New York State hospitals. That study was completed and publicly reported in 1989, just as Congress was creating two additional Quality of Care and Patient Safety agencies, and that number of agencies would be increased to five during, first the Clinton, and later the Obama Administrations. Those Federal Agencies would become like the Sun that multiple other private and professional organizations would revolve around and collaborate with.

What's my point? This vast army of experts have been working their magic now for over 3 decades prior to COVID while receiving billions of dollars from Congress, and no one can identify any clearly definable improvement in making hospital patient care safer. It has all been a gigantic fraud, and every elected decision-maker at Federal and State level has ignored this tragedy that has resulted in the level of needless hospital deaths being unchanged for those 3 decades prior to COVID.

Case in point: House Oversight Committee

Our mission statement is to ensure the efficiency, effectiveness, and accountability of the federal government and all its agencies. We provide a check and balance on the role and power of Washington and a voice to the people it serves.

I doubt any member of the House Oversight Committee, and their many staff members, could even begin to provide a reasonably accurate description of those 5 Quality of Care and Patient Safety agencies despite all of the billions of dollars they have been receiving beginning in 1970. Agency for Healthcare Research and Quality (AHRQ) was created in 1989 and bills itself as; the lead Federal agency charged with improving the safety and quality of healthcare for all Americans. When Dr. Makary claimed that Medical Errors are the third leading cause of deaths in the U.S. 27 years later, they remained silent. But more on the utter failure of those well-funded federal agencies will begin.

Forest Gump said, "Stupid is as stupid does.", and Congress, and all 50 state governors and legislatures have consistently ignored the overwhelming evidence of major problems within every level of the Healthcare Delivery System. Selective stupidity has reigned supreme while clothe in monumental indifference.

A multitude of those identified as the major leaders of the various agencies and organizations are treated like Rock Stars at the many conferences and gatherings held annually. Yet this well-established army of experts seems to exist in their own private world because few people in the real world would be capable of recognizing their names. I know that to be true because I once asked the members of the Board of the largest Healthcare System in South Carolina to take such a name-recognition test, and each Board member failed that test completely. Here you have several Board members who are the decision-makers for the largest healthcare system in their state, and they are unable to recognize the names of the key persons who have been claiming to be improving the Quality of Care and Patient Safety in every hospital in the Nation. I found the results of that exercise to be frightening, but I suspect such information will fall on deaf ears.

The Healthcare Delivery System, and its long-standing, inherent problems are real, and clearly evident IF, and only if that critical issue can begin to receive the consideration it so desperately deserves and should demand. So, why do I feel I might be capable of supplying the necessary boost to elevate that issue to public interest?

Whistleblowers typically appear out of nowhere, and as a red-neck dentist who can claim no degree of recognition anywhere seems to fit my starting-point. Yet, I feel I can justify my qualification as a healthcare whistleblower by my books, and my past accomplishments, and beginning with Agnes in Madison WI.

My being the person who established the first major-surgical mini-residency of any surgical specialty in the Nation in 1970 and have that accomplishment to be replicated multiple times by multiple established oral surgery training programs is a feat that I believe would have been far more newsworthy if it had taken place in any of the many medical surgical training programs. Over 50 years ago I was able to do something that had never been done before, and that was worthy of being repeated should provide me with some degree of consideration.

I may also be the only person who forced every level of medical staff leadership, and hospital administration, and governing board to perform documented peer review of a patient's negligible care, and then certify such negligent care to be that hospital medical staff's newly accepted standard of care for future patients with similar injuries. I suspect but have no way to prove if my efforts to force complete patient-care peer review at every level of authority in not only one hospital, but also within a religious-based healthcare system of 14 hospitals was not only one-of-a-kind, but possibly the only such exercise in complete medical peer review ever accomplished. That episode should be worthy of careful study, particularly since I retain all the official documents, but I cannot imagine that the AMA and American Hospital Association (AHA) would ever be interested in such a review. Agnes' story is worthy of being included in any history of medical care, but I doubt if such a review will ever take place. Organized Medicine has no real interest in visiting the Dark Side of their Profession, but it will continue to be impossible to ever begin even to create a better healthcare system without complete understanding of that Dark Side, and the 3 decades long efforts to improve Patient Safety within that "System" prior to COVID. And there is no better place to begin than with the one person who personifies those efforts.

Dr. Lucian Leape
Father of Patient Safety

Dr. Lucian Leape (pronounced Leap) practiced pediatric surgery for two decades prior to redirecting his medical experience to healthcare policy in general, and the efforts to begin to better understand quality of care and patient safety issues in mid-1980, just as others were doing the same. And there is no better way to describe Dr. Leape's participation in those efforts that eventually led his efforts to qualify him to be recognized as the Father of Patient Safety than to let him speak for himself.

Making Healthcare Safe
The Story of the Patient Safety Movement
Lucian L. Leape, MD

Making Healthcare Safe first appeared as an open access publication in 2021, and I was fortunately able to capture that manuscript on my computer, and while it is a valuable resource for obtaining a far better understanding of those efforts to improve patient safety, it is also important to state that Dr.

Leape's contribution to that better understanding is clearly stated to be limited to the period from 1987 to 2015, thereby failing to include any of those efforts that took place during the last 5 years of those efforts prior to COVID. Therefore, Dr. Leape's retirement from that vast army of experts, and his being the "Father" of those efforts for at least two decades as of 2015, did not result in any pause of those efforts continuing.

The point here is that Dr. Leape's Making Healthcare Safe, The Story of the Patient Safety Movement is his effort to present those 3 decades of efforts as though the current Healthcare Delivery System had truly become far safer for patients in 2015 than it had been when he first joined those efforts in the mid-1980s. Nothing could be further from the truth, and later comments by other healthcare experts will demonstrate that fallacy. But, since Dr. Leape's manuscript was an open access publication, it is only fair to permit him to speak for himself.

Foreword

This book is an invaluable and unique account of the evolution of the evidence, concern, activities, and structures that inform the world's current understanding of how patients are injured too often by the care that is intended to help them and what can and should be done about that. For a topic of such enormous gravity, involving life-or-death consequences every year for tens of thousands of people in the USA, alone, and many hundreds of thousands globally, this story is remarkably recent. The modern scientific foundations for safety in every sector of human endeavor were laid first no earlier than the mid-twentieth century, and the application of those sciences to medical care, with just a few, slender exceptions, began only in the mid-1980s, barely 40 years ago as of this writing.

Note, too, that the journey to patient safety has, in actuality, barely begun. Lucian and his colleagues advocating for safer care, I among them, are all too aware of how incomplete the victory is. To our chagrin, and to the disadvantaged millions of patients and families, improving safety still lacks the strategic centering it ought to have in the health care organizations both public and private. Governments around the world still generally lack agencies and individuals responsible for assuring and nurturing safety systems and safety results. Professional training still barely mentions the topic, and the scientific armamentarium for safe systems is almost nowhere taught to the physicians, nurses, and health care managers of tomorrow. No one escapes medical school without studying the Krebs cycle and hearing about the discovery of insulin; but almost all will graduate without 1 minute of learning about human error or a single encounter with the work of James Reason.

As a result, the toll of error and injury to patients continues to be massive. In 2018, three important reports on defects in quality in global health care were published, one ("Crossing the Global Quality Chasm") from the National Academies of Sciences, Engineering, and Medicine in the USA, one from The Lancet Commission on High-Quality Health Systems in the Sustainable Development Goals Era, and one ("Delivering

Quality Health Services: A Global Imperative for Universal Health Coverage") from the World Health Organization,

OECD, and the World Bank. Though carried out separately, these reports each estimated that over five million deaths a year in the world can be attributed to defects in the quality of health care. Problems in patient safety are high among those causes. So, the story told in this book, as compelling as it is, will be but Chapter One of the longer-term saga of the patient safety movement. The work of safety improvement, indeed, is hardly begun. No one hopes more than does Lucian Leape that the next book will be able to recount vast successes not yet in our hands.

Donald M. Berwick, Institute for Healthcare Improvement, Boston, MA, USA.

Dr. Berwick's Foreword was written in 2021, and one line speaks volumes, "As a result, the toll of error and injury to patients continues to be massive." That quote clearly summarizes the actual results of 3 decades of efforts by that vast army of quality-of-care experts; Abject Failure! It has all been a lie. Five Federal Agencies, surrounded by many, many professional, and private entities, all seeking to make Your & Your Loved One's Healthcare Delivery System safer, and they have NOTHING to show for all their efforts.

More strange is that I have been saying for the past several years that;

I know Why, and I know How the current HCDS is, and has always been broken, but more importantly, I know How to begin to create a 21st century HCDS, and no one has shown even the slightest interest in what I might have to offer.

But first, I say it has all been a lie, because there is NO discernable evidence to contradict my assertion. Doctors dominate the quality-of-care army of experts, and one of Dr. Leape's first statements will provide a basic understanding of why everything said by those experts for over 3 decades was based upon that edict.

"As we will see with the AMA later, anything that might possibly make doctors look bad was unacceptable." (Chapter 1, page 5)

That profound recognition is the root cause of why NO discernable improvement has been made in the efforts to improve the quality of care and patient safety, and despite all of the documented efforts to do so. And that is why I believe Agnes' story, and my documented efforts to force medical peer review is relevant today. The target is to make medical care safer, but no one is allowed to speak or write anything that might reflect poorly on doctors. And that is my basis for saying that all those efforts for over 3 decades prior to COVID can be proven to be a LIE. And that is why, in my third book, FIND THE BLACK BOX, PREVENT NEEDLESS HOSPITAL DEATHS, self-published in 2013 I said that in my opinion, Dr. Lucian Leape was the Father of a Miscarriage.

The following is two pages of notes I took as I read Dr. Leape's open access manuscript. Each page notes a comment or subject that I feel I would be able to discuss in detail, and in most I feel I could offer strong support to refute.

Making Healthcare Safe

The Story of the Patient Safety Movement
Lucian Leape, MD 2021

Foreword—Donald M. Berwick, MD
Institute for Healthcare Improvement

Page VII. For Lucian Leape, it has meant, not just witnessing the historic birth of the health care patient safety movement, but, arguably, creating it. My response to that is NONSENSE!

Page X. Note, too, that the journey to patient safety has barely begun. Lucian and his colleagues advocating for safer care, I among them, are all too aware of how incomplete the victory is. To our chagrin, and to the disadvantage of millions of patients and families, improving safety still lacks the strategic centering it ought to have in the health care organizations both public and private. I CAN PROVIDE WHAT IS MISSING!

Preface

Page XIII. The story runs roughly from 1987 to 2015.

Page 5. As we will see with the AMA later, anything that might possibly make doctors look bad was unacceptable.

Page 7. States required hospitals to report deaths but rarely investigated their causes. The Joint Commission asked hospitals to report "sentinel events" (serious injuries), but few hospitals did... Medical injury was largely invisible, and hospitals and doctor liked it that way.

Page 13. Reviewers would not "see" events that hadn't happened! On balance, we believed that our rates, shocking as they were, *underestimated* the true extent of harm. In fact, later studies would bear that out.

Page 14. NEJM: Brennan & Leape, two articles in 1991. But interest in the study faded quickly.

Page 17. "Don't go there>" Howard Hiatt and Troy Brennan were emphatic: investigating medical error and writing about it would bring the wrath of the medical profession down on my head... How could we not act?

Page 18. I took my search strategy to the librarian and asked for help. She thought the strategy was fine but asked if had looked in the social sciences or engineering literature. It hadn't occurred to me.

James Reason, of the University of Manchester, UL, is without doubt the person who has contributed the most to the understanding of the causes and prevention of errors. His book, *Human Error* (1990), is the "Bible" of error theory.

Page 20. The more I read, the more excited I got about the relevance of this knowledge to what we needed to do to reduce iatrogenic harm. I assumed that, like me, very few doctors, nurses, or other healthcare workers had any knowledge of this body of thought. It seemed inescapably clear that healthcare needed to take a systems approach to medical errors. (1988)

We needed to stop punishing individuals for their errors since almost all of them were beyond their control, and we had to begin to change the faulty systems that "set them up" to make mistakes. We needed to design errors out of the system. I had no doubt we could do that.

Page 24. I ended the paper with a summary that was more prophetic than I realized at the time. "But it is apparent that the most fundamental change that will be needed if hospitals are to make meaningful progress in error reduction is a cultural one.

Page 45. 1996 was the year that patient safety began.

Page 50. A surprise announcement by Nancy Dickey, the incoming chairman of the AMA Board, that the AMA was founding and funding a National Patient Safety Foundation.

Page 51. "Annenberg," as we all later called the first conference, was the birthplace of patient safety—in the USA and, truly, in the world.

Page 69. Dr. Berwick, at a chance meeting with Paul Batalden, who introduced him to the work of W. Edwards Deming.

Page 70. Dr. Berwick found Deming's work on quality management in industry fascinating. ****

Page 71. Berwick wrote up his ideas about how these concepts could be applied in healthcare in a NEJM article (1989. [My note: This led Dr. Berwick, and 2 Co-Authors to write a book, *Curing Healthcare* in 1990.]

Page 79. Dr. Peter Pronovost dramatically demonstrated its effectiveness in reducing central line catheter-associated infections in 2004.

Page 83. It is impossible to overstate the impact of IHI on quality of healthcare and patient safety. Under the inspired, skilled, and impassioned leadership of Don Berwick, IHI established a corporate model that has yielded a never-ending stream of innovative and effective methods to improve care and reduce harm.

Page 127. On July 7, 1998, I received an invitation from the Institute of Medicine (IOM) to become a member of the Committee on Quality of Health Care in America.

[**My Note:** *Chapter 9, pp 127-139 is a documentation of multiple experts, with the best of intentions, demonstrating Einstein's definition of insanity. None of those "experts" can provide any evidence of their having the ability to describe, in detail, the enormous, complex, Healthcare Delivery System (doctors & hospitals) they claim to be seeking to improve, and over two decades after this "Report", there is still NO evidence any substantial improvement in the Quality of Care and Patient Safety has ever taken place. In fact, To Err Is Human, and the other Reports" (Books) that rapidly followed) have proved to be colossal failures, despite all the undeserved praise given.]*

Page 143. Agency for Healthcare Policy and Research (AHCPR), now Agency for Healthcare Research and Quality (AHRQ) was first commissioned in 1989.

Page 146. Congress passed the Healthcare Research and Quality Act in 1999.

Page 147. The scope was breathtaking. Healthcare had never seen anything like it. Shalala asked Eisenberg to brief the president on the report. When he did, he found that Clinton had not only read the entire report but understood it. He asked John whether it was possible, as the IOM report challenged, for healthcare to reduce preventable deaths by 50% in 5 years. John said yes, or even in 2 years or 1 year—*because hospitals would manipulate their measures to make it appear that happened.* (emphasis mine)

Page 148. Carolyn Clancy took over as director and expanded AHRQ's activities and influence as the major force advancing patient safety.

Page 151. Evidence-Based Practices. AHRQ commissioned an Evidence-Based Practices group at the Un. Of Cal. At San Francisco led by Bob Wachter and Kaveh Shojania to review the evidence and report in 6 months.

Page 155. in 2005 Congress established Patient Safety Organizations (PSOs).

Page 156. As Gray observed, AHRQ's political problems are three-dimensional. [A must read]

Page 157. To health policy experts, it seems obvious that AHRQ should become an institute as part of NIH, with an annual funding at $1-2 billion level, which is less than that currently provided for several institutes for conditions that affect far fewer people and cause far fewer deaths.

Pages 159-62. Setting Standards" The National Quality Forum: Sept. 1, 1999.

Page 164. Serious Reportable Events

Page 171. At the end of 2005, Kizer stepped down, and Janet Corrigan took over as president.

Page 174. Conflict of Interest Scandal: Charles Denham

Page 176. Appendix 11.1: Serious Reportable Events Steering Committee: St. Mary Jean Ryan, FSM, President, SSM Healthcare, St. Louis, MO. [a criminal organization in 1979 in Madison WI—I know the facts.]

Chapter 12 Enforcing Standards: The Joint Commission

Page 185. The JC has been for many years the principal driver of healthcare quality. GAG!

Page 188. The Agenda for Change–1986

Page 189. Paul Batalden and Don Berwick had studied under Deming...

Page 191. Focus on Patient Safety: Sentinel Events–1995, the death of Betsy Lehman in Boston.

Page 231. Chapter 15 Just Do It: The Surgical Checklist

Page 262. The Journal of Patient Safety–Denham again.

Part IV Creating a Culture of Safety
Chapter 22 Make No Little Plans: The Lucian Leape Institute

Page 372. Paul Gluck, Immediate past chair of NPSF Board of Directors.

Some may consider my critical interpretation of Dr. Leape's epic history of patient safety efforts during his active participation in those efforts to be unkind, but one must remember that Dr. Leape was anointed with the title of *Father of Patient Safety*, his book only covers those efforts between 1987 and 2015, and even Dr. Berwick admitted in 2021.,

> *"As a result, the toll of error and injury to patients continues to be massive."*

And only one year later recognition of a true assessment of patient safety in America was publicly acknowledged.

Medical Errors are the 3rd leading cause of deaths in the U.S. behind heart disease and cancer. Marty Makary, MD, and Michael Daniel, 2016

One year after the period covered in Dr. Leape's book, Making Healthcare Safe ends, other healthcare policy experts appear to recognize what should have long been recognized; all the efforts of that vast army of quality-of-care experts have been worthless. Why? Medical errors are caused by doctors, but those quality-of-care experts were never allowed to say anything "bad" about doctors, and each component of that vast army is typically led by doctors.

Even more troubling is the fact that not an eye blinked in Washington DC, and not an eye blinked in any of the fifty state capitals in response to that assertion, and I do not understand that. Does Selective Stupidity come to mind?

Mistreated, why we think we're getting good health care–and why we're usually WRONG.

Robert Pearl, MD, 2017. As noted throughout Mistreated, the current health care system is broken. It most closely resembles a nineteenth-century cottage industry. (Page 224)

While Dr. Leape was writing his Making Healthcare Safe sanitized history of efforts to improve patient safety during the 28-year period covered by his book, other healthcare experts were providing the public with a far different, and more accurate assessment of Your & Your Loved One's Healthcare Delivery System. The current system is broken, it has always been broken, and there are clear reasons why. But Selective Stupidity ignores those clear facts.

I must take exception to his exaggerated analogy likening the current system to a 19th century (1800-1899) cottage industry. Pasteur established the Germ Theory late in the 19th century, and finally began to try to convince doctors that they had been killing many of their patients due to "no-seeums" that they, the doctors, had been passing on to their patients unknowingly. Pasteur opened the door to Modern Medicine. Our Presidents, Congresses, State Governors, and Legislators created the current, ill-organized HCDS on their collective own. But, back to Dr. Makary, and his ground-breaking contribution to every attempt to raise the alarm that all the past efforts to improve patient safety had merely been doctors leading those efforts while ignoring the fact that doctors are the root-cause of those patient safety issues.

Early in the morning, on a mid-November Saturday in 2012, I began reading my Wall Street Journal first on the D-section front page, and there I saw a picture of the book cover, and a book review of.

UNACCOUNTABLE, What Hospitals Won't Tell You and How Transparency Can Revolutionize Health Care, Marty Makary, MD, 2012

Dr. Makary's book is, in my opinion, the first book that took readers further behind the black curtain of the medical profession than ever before. His book was featured on the front page of the Wall Street Journal Saturday edition D section in mid-November 2012. I read that review, went to Barnes & Noble and purchased a copy that day, and when I finished reading his book, I said; "I have to write another book." *FIND THE BLACK BOX,* my 3rd book was self-published in late summer, 2013, but more about Dr. Makary's book.

Dr. Makary graciously permitted me to quote excerpts of his book into my book, and I reprint some of those excerpts here to demonstrate that I am not the only healthcare professional who is deeply concerned with the shortcomings of the medical, and equally so in my case, the dental profession.

Dr. Makary Excerpts from Unaccountable

But then it hit me: A hospital is no longer the community pillar I knew growing up, with its altruistic mission guiding its decisions. Hospitals have merged and transformed into giant corporations with little accountability—and they like it that way.

In 2010, a Harvard study published in the prestigious New England Journal of Medicine reported a finding well-known to medical professionals: as many as 25% of all patients are harmed by medical mistakes. What's even less known to the public is that over the past ten years, error rates have not come down, despite numerous efforts to make medical care safer.

Dr. Lucian Leape, at a national surgeon's conference opened the gathering's keynote speech by looking out over the audience of thousands and asking the doctors to "raise your hand if you know of a physician you work with who should not be practicing because he or she is dangerous." Every hand went up. Incredulous at this response, I took to asking the same question whenever I spoke at conferences. And I always got the same response. Every doctor knows about this problem—but few talk about it. Every day, people are injured or killed by medical mistake that might have been prevented with a modicum of adherence to standardize guidelines. The silence about the problem has paralyzed efforts to address it—until now. Medicine is its own culture. It has its own language, ethos, and code of justice. Doctors swear to do no harm. But on the job, they soon absorb another unspoken rule: to overlook malpractice in their colleagues.

We all know the health care system is broken, burdens our families, businesses, and national debt. It needs common-sense reform.

There were other, more powerful ways I was "educated" on the code of silence. Once in a hospital peer-review conference, I witnessed the futility of a brave doctors speaking up to condemn another doctor's careless decision to operate when the operation didn't meet criteria. The doctor at fault gave a justification that a courtroom would believe, but we all knew it was not true. It was a rare spectacle, yet nothing came out of it, except that the brave doctor who spoke up became a marked man. Throughout my training I witnessed several doctors run out of town because their honesty and outspokenness begin to poke the bear. In many ways, direct and indirect, I was taught that the code of silence was part of being a doctor.

Unlike aviation, hundreds of thousands of lives are lost each year due to preventable mistakes by doctors.

Seeking accurate ways to measure patient outcomes has long been the holy grail of health care reform, the starting point for fixing our broken health care system.

As I listened to Dr. Leape talk about secret addictions and other common impairments, I realized that he wasn't just talking about doctors who simply have poor skills or bad judgment. This was an entirely different problem. He was talking about doctors affected by dependence problems and other physical and mental impairments. That's when the problem of impaired physicians struck me as nothing less than a public health crisis. I did some more math. If, say, only 2% of the nation's one million doctors are seriously impaired by drugs, alcohol abuse, or other major impairments (and most experts agree that 2% is a low estimate), that means twenty thousand impaired doctors are practicing medicine. I asked, "What can be done about these few bad apples affecting so many people?" Dr. Leape smiled, and said, "The state medical boards take care of that."

Yet there are also grossly impaired physicians, doctors with horrible skills, hazardous judgment, ulterior motive motives, or who suffer from substance-abuse or other problems that make them dangerous. Society ought to be able to deal with this better, not sweep it all under the rug. Doctoring is a stressful profession with easy access to drugs, so it's no mystery why doctors have substance abuse problems. In fact, rates of serious substance abuse and psychiatric disease among doctors are higher than that of other professions with similar educational background in socio-economic status.

However, based on Halsted's life and what I've seen in my career, I agree with others that 2% is a drastic understatement of the true incidence of impaired physicians.

One time, right after this notoriously bad surgeons run of six deaths, my friend was administrating anesthesia for him. In front of all the operating room nurses and technicians, the patient asked my friend before going off to sleep, "Is my surgeon a good surgeon?" The operating room staff froze as their eyes popped out of their heads. They stared at my friend to see how he would deal with the direct question. "He's one of the four best heart surgeons we have here", he said with a smile. Luckily for my friend, the patient didn't follow up with, "And how many heart surgeons do you have here?"

Having inside knowledge about a risky doctor while trying to comfort his patient in preparation for surgery is a dilemma every health care provider knows all too well. I asked my friend if he ever thought about reporting this surgeon to someone. He laughed and asked, "Like who?"

The hospital administration loved this young heart surgeon, who was making a financial killing (pardon the pun) off his work. The senior partners were very protective of him as the youngest member of their group—after all, he took most of their weekend calls for them. He covered their holiday shifts and happily tended to whatever the senior surgeons did not like to do, such as operating on their obese patients for them. They cut the young doc tremendous slack whenever his complications were discussed at a peer-review conference, saying a patient's death was attributable to some extenuating patient circumstances. (That's right, they'd blame the victim.)

Such internal peer reviews are a little like the Russian parliament under Stalin. No matter how much discussion there is, the result seems foreordained. At these internal peer review conferences, complicated cases are reduced to biased two-to-three-minute summaries, and doctors who might raise probing questions understand they can pay a heavy price for challenging their peers.

Doctors and nurses know of docs who are reckless, but it takes moving a mountain to do something about it. Not reporting incompetence among peers is part of medical culture and has been for centuries. Medicine is poorly policed.

How about the national doctor's associations? Can they police their own time? As a member of several, only once have

I ever heard of a program that tried to address impaired physicians, and that effort never picked up steam. After asking around, it became clear that the only time that a doctor's association would ever consider acting against the doctor was if a state medical board had already done so. Hungry to grow their membership and collect annual dues, doctors' associations are historically passive when it comes to policing doctors (the AMA is actively recruiting to increase its membership, which is now declined to 15% of US doctors; membership cost $420 a year). Policing doctors is a job so messy no one wants to do it.

So, who is in charge of policing medical care in America?

Every organization, institution, medical Association, and hospital administrator that have I have asked has told me that policing physicians is the real responsibility of state medical boards. So, let's examine the role of state medical boards in American medicine.

State Medical Boards

Consider California. The Medical Board of California, like all others is responsible for licensing and disciplining physicians. On three different audits conducted during the 1980s, the California auto to general found that the board wasn't doing its job. Apart from that announcement, no further action was taken. The board went 18 years without another audit until 2003, when University of San Diego Law School Professor Julie D'Angelo Fellmeth became the medical board enforcement monitor. Then she blew a whistle. Testifying to a Senate committee in 2008 after years of trying to sound alarms, she said the Medical Board of California "routinely failed to promptly remove from work physician participants who tested positive for prohibited substances." The board had five out of five failed audit audits. Julie D'Angelo Fellmeth was let go. The Medical Board of California then went on doing whatever it does about impaired physicians, which is to say, not much.

Impaired physicians are a small minority of doctors who are very destructive and difficult to police. Knowingly or unknowingly, they cause a lot of harm. State medical boards are sometimes aware of them but look the other way. Standards for doctors are local and vary widely state by state.

Nearly every doctor can name a doctor who needs to retire but won't—impaired doctors in their 90's who refused to leave the office even when they are no longer being paid. Why do we have this problem? The reason is there are no rules.

I can legally do anything. In fact, some varicose-vein removal centers in the United States are run by former OB/GYN doctors and others by psychiatrists; they were doctors looking to do something different and took a weekend course to learn how to do it. Putting aside how I get paid; I can do whatever I want in medicine with little to no accountability.

Being in the medical-errors field has decreased my threshold for shock. A New England Journal of Medicine study concluded that as many as 25% of all hospitalized patients will experience a preventable medical error of some kind. Almost everyone I talk to has a story about a friend or family member who was hurt, disfigured, are killed by medical mistake. Even me.

My research partner, Peter Pronovost, lost his father due to a medical error when Peter was in medical school. My medical partner, Dr. Patrick O'Kolo, lost his younger sister due to a medical error. My best friend's mom had her breast removed unnecessarily because she was mistakenly told she had stage-three breast cancer. After her procedure, her doctors told her the original report had a mistake—she had only had stage one and hadn't needed a breast removal after all. My grandfather died at age 60 from a condition called urosepsis, a preventable infection following a surgery he didn't even need. My brother has a wide scar on his back from his stitches popping open after a skin mole was removed; he thinks it was unavoidable bad luck, but I can tell the surgeon used stitches too weak to hold the skin together. My cousin worked with a cardiac surgeon and witness countless deaths from an impaired physician. I myself was misdiagnosed with a knee problem in medical school.

Listening to Peter and many friends who have similar stories, I realize that the patent these patients suffered not just from their botched treatments but from the knowledge that their misfortune need never have happened. For them, talking about medical mistakes is part of their healing. But our system wants to sweep them under the rug and keep them quiet. I sometimes hear egregious stories from people who preface their accounts with, "Please keep this just between you and may, because I signed a waiver saying that I would never talk about this." When a doctor or hospital does harm a patient, this settlement offer from the hospital often contains a confidentiality clause (a.k.a. "a gag rule"). In fact, in any case of gross neglect, hospital lawyers will aggressively pursue victims or their surviving family to settle out-of-court quickly in order to stem off a malpractice suit—provided they agree never to speak about what happened, even if one has been disfigured, maimed, or killed.

In order to get a handle on the widespread epidemic of medical mistakes, we need more conversation about them, not less.

There are bad doctors and impaired doctors, but the problem of doctors making repeated avoidable mistakes is a management problem.

Every health services researcher knows errors are common. Medical mistakes are not only far more common than they should be—they are a devastating cost burden on our health care system.

Patients under his care suffered because of these communication breakdowns. All this renegade needed was someone higher up the food chain—somebody with authority over his career—to take him aside and tell him to correct his attitude toward his coworkers. That never happened. He continued to terrorize his staff to the detriment of his patients.

How can we ensure accountability across the field of health care? In principle, most doctors and most hospital administrators agree that accountability is a good thing. But when it comes to being accountable themselves, they are often less enthusiastic. This is only human nature. Taking the extra effort to follow procedures meticulously or keep records of our performance can seem burdensome. And reducing your own accountability can protect your reputation and cover-up sins. You are freer to do what you want without having to bother about how other people will react. But a lack of accountability can alienate those who serve and fuel distrust. Moreover, knowing your accountable improves your performance.

Medicine is an institution as old as humanity. Its traditions are as hierarchical as those of the royals. And for centuries, doctors have enhanced their authority with mystery, keeping the workings of their profession opaque. But I am convinced that the new generation of doctors is poised to usher in a revolution of transparency, open-mindedness, and honesty. This generational shift may be just what is needed for medicine to end the secrecy that has historically permeated our profession. With younger doctors taking the lead, the culture is ripe for transformation if we can capitalize on this moment and push for reform from within.

My Response: Dr. Makary's book takes the reader behind the curtain, and into the inter-workings of hospital medical staffs, and particularly, teaching hospital medical staffs, and his one-word title speaks volumes regarding the true status of patient safety throughout the history of our nation's healthcare delivery system. When you put the word unaccountable with Dr. Leape's admission, as we will see with the AMA later, anything that might possibly make doctors look bad was unacceptable. Those are the reasons why all those 3 decades of promises to make healthcare safer, while only actually merely providing lip-service, it all begins to make sense. There is no evidence that real improvement in protecting patients from negligent care has been effectively established throughout that "system" that has long been recognized to be a non-system. One should particularly notice Dr. Makary's recognition of the destructive nature of the Code of Silence. All the failures of the medical profession's responsibilities to protect the public from unqualified doctors are rooted in the Code of Silence.

I couldn't stop showcasing so many of his quotes because they all mirror what I have been trying to present to any interested persons, decision-makers, and non-decision-makers, about what is missing, and has always been missing in our Health Care Delivery System.

The major difference between Dr. Makary's message and mine is that he sees the Problem, while I see both the Problem and the Solution. Hopefully, Dr. Makary is right, and the "culture" within the Medical Profession and the Hospital Administration Profession is changing and becoming more receptive to considering fundamental change. Unfortunately, I am not as optimistic because I see no evidence of a desire, or even a recognition for a need to fundamentally change the direction of current efforts anywhere in the Quality of Health Care Experts' literature.

Sue or Forget It, and the response it receives from within the Quality of Health Care Army, when coupled with Dr. Makary's well-received UNACCOUNTABLE and its quest for fundamental change, should indicate if the components of our current Health Care Delivery System are truly ready, willing, and able to confront these issues openly and in a meaningful manner.

While Agnes' story clearly demonstrates the all too typical failure of professional responsibility for harmed patients by both at the hospital medical staff level, and the hospital administration, there was also a clear demonstration of unprofessional behavior by another, major component of Organized Medicine.

Pause

I feel I must pause here, and try to put the contents, and intent of this book in proper perspective. I am attempting to become the Healthcare Whistleblower by identifying, and clarifying what has always been missing in the decades-long efforts and promises to make Your & Your Lover One's Healthcare Delivery System (doctors & hospitals) far safer, and how all of those efforts have been misguided, and ineffective.

I repeat what I said earlier, Dr. Jeffrey Wigand achieved national prominence in 1995 when he became the tobacco industry's highest ranking former executive to finally begin to tell the truth about the health effects of smoking, and what the top leaders of that industry had always known. I am trying to do the same regarding the long-standing failures on how to begin to make the delivery of healthcare far safer.

Dr. Wigand was able to provide overwhelming evidence of all that the leaders of the tobacco industry had long known but had kept secret. There is over-whelming evidence, clearly available to demonstrate what has always been missing in the efforts to make the delivery of healthcare far safer, and there has been no Dr. Wigands within the Quality of Care and Patient Safety Movement willing to step forward and begin to tell the truth, that is until now. I seek to be the Dr. Wigand of Healthcare, and I can only do that by demonstrating how all of those current and past experts have been praising their decades of efforts of abject failure.

One can assume that the ideal person to guide such a demonstration would be Dr. Lucian Leape, Father of Patient Safety, and his recent 28-year historical timeline of his participation in the efforts and promises to make the delivery of healthcare safer as recorded in his Making Healthcare Safe, The Story of the Patient Safety Movement. And since his book was a free download, I will use excerpts from his book in order to allow him to speak for himself. But first, his recollections of the Patient Safety efforts between 1987 and 2015 should be put into proper perspective.

President Johnson and Congress created Medicare and Medicaid in the mid-1960s. and it rapidly became clear that hospitals seeking to receive funds from those new Federal sources of revenue would require some means of certification of each hospital's worthiness to participate in those programs. Joint Commission (an arm of Organized Medicine) was chosen, along with the American Osteopathic Association (AOA) who demanded that they be permitted to certify Osteopathic hospitals, and such was granted. It is important to acknowledge that various elements of Organized Medicine had been certifying the quality of care provided by hospital medical staffs for over two decades prior to the beginning of the events described by Dr. Leape. The following will consist of excerpts taken from Making Healthcare Safe as he (Dr. Leape) describes a series of significant events during that 28-year period and includes my comments at the end of each separate segment. The purpose of combining Dr. Leape's description of those events, and my critique of the true value of any possible contribution those separate events might have made in making the delivery of healthcare safer are included to demonstrate, in my opinion, that all of the efforts to improve the quality of care and patient safety for over three decades before COVID have proven to be Abject Failures, and Dr. Leape has been the Father of a monumental miscarriage. But the reader must judge for themselves, because the true subject to this book is Your & Your Loved One's Healthcare Delivery System (doctors & hospitals), and as a whistleblower, my purpose is to attempt to prove that all those past efforts have been valueless. So, we begin with Dr. Leape's first leap into the first big effort to try to determine the extent of *Adverse Events* (AE) in hospital patient care.

Making Healthcare Safe (excerpts)

And no one had any idea of the costs of medical injury—financial, physical, and emotional: not just the costs of continuing medical treatment, but of lost wages, childcare, home assistance, and long-term disability. Reflecting on all of this, Howard Hiatt, dean of the Harvard School of Public Health (HSPH), and his good friend, James Vorenberg, dean of the Harvard Law School, conceived of the idea of doing a study to answer these questions. What were the costs of medical injury? How much of it was due to negligence? How successfully did the liability insurance system meet its purported objectives of compensating the injured and deterring bad practice? Did the risk of being sued make doctors more careful and thus reduce the likelihood of patients being harmed? Did the system fairly compensate those who were harmed? Some experts had expressed interest in no-fault insurance that would pay for all the costs of injury for all patients, irrespective of negligence. Would such a scheme be an economically feasible alternative to litigation? Surely among the faculty of their two schools, they reasoned, there should be enough brainpower to answer these questions and perhaps even develop a better solution. The place to start, they thought, was with the facts. How many people were harmed by medical treatment in hospitals? What percentage was caused by errors? By negligence? Of those harmed by negligent care, how many sued? What were the costs of medical injury—not just for those harmed by bad care, but for all patients, including those who suffered nonpreventable injuries? How were these costs paid for? All was unknown. All was potentially knowable. With colleagues, they designed a study to get this information. They used as a model a 1978 study by Don Harper Mills of "potentially compensable events" (PCEs): medical injuries for which a jury might award.

Howard's first thought was to seek the approval of the Massachusetts Medical Society, so he approached the president of the society, whom he knew. She thought it was a very bad idea! As we will see with the AMA later, anything that might possibly make doctors look bad was unacceptable. Similarly, Howard found no "takers" among the various private foundations or governmental authorities in Massachusetts. But suddenly, there was interest in New York. Howard described the plan to his friend Alfred Gellhorn, who introduced him to the Commissioner of Health in New York State, David Axelrod, whose response was quite positive. Axelrod took him to meet Governor Mario Cuomo, who said, "We've been looking for you! When can you get started?" Cuomo was struggling with state spending for medical liability claims that was substantial and increasing. Would the Harvard team be willing to do it in New York State? They were delighted to do so—New York's large size and diversity would make the results more credible. When told how much it would cost, Cuomo commented that he expected it to be several times that amount, and he readily authorized an appropriation of $3.2 million for the study. The Robert Wood Johnson Foundation contributed an additional $250,000.

Hiatt led the research team. Troy Brennan and Nan Laird led the study design. Troy was just finishing his chief residency in medicine at the Massachusetts General Hospital, but he was uniquely qualified for this study. A Rhodes scholar, he was an honors MD and MPH graduate of Yale Medical School, while simultaneously receiving his JD from Yale Law School. Nan Laird was a professor of statistics, later department chair, at the Harvard School of Public Health.

The team was about 6 months into the study when, in the spring of 1987, Howard Hiatt approached me to determine my interest in joining them. After 20 years in academic pediatric surgery, I wanted to work in health policy and was finishing a year as a fellow at RAND studying epidemiology, statistics, and health policy in preparation for my new career. At RAND I had become involved in several studies of overuse of healthcare services and was leading a study of underuse. I was returning to Boston and looking for additional opportunities in my new career.

We sought a neutral term that captured all events and to which we could apply a judgment of negligence when indicated. We finally settled on "adverse event." We spent many hours debating its exact definition and ultimately agreed on "an unintended injury that was caused by medical management rather than the patient's underlying disease." The important point was to distinguish harm caused by treatment from harm caused by disease, independent of whether there was an error or negligence. We knew that making this judgment would be difficult for doctors, as it indeed proved to be. Physicians are very sensitive to any implication that their performance is deficient in any way. Complications were considered either "preventable," which meant someone was to blame, or unpreventable. Most were put in the latter category, which included certain types of complications that everyone knew occasionally happened and were thought to be unavoidable and therefore no one's fault, as well as the occasional unanticipated outcome that seemed to come out of the blue. Our hope was that reviewers could view "adverse event" as a neutral term.

The most common source of injury caused by treatment in the hospital, of course, is a surgical operation, so it was necessary to distinguish this form of planned harm from that due to errors or other failures. Use of the word "unintended" resolved that problem. We struggled unsuccessfully to devise a reliable way to measure psychological harm, despite its obvious importance, so we restricted our study to physical harm. For "error," we used Reason's definition: "The failure of a planned action to be completed as intended or the use of a wrong plan to achieve an aim." For "negligence," we used the standard accepted legal definition: "Failure to meet the standard of care." The plan was to obtain data by reviewing medical records of hospitalized patients. We would focus on adverse events that could potentially trigger a malpractice suit.

Finding and training physicians to review the records was more difficult. With help from the NY Department of Health and strong support from the NY State Medical Society, we identified and recruited board-certified internists and surgeons in each of the fifty-one towns where our study hospitals were. To minimize conflicts of interest, we required that these physicians not be on the staff or have admitting privileges at the hospital whose records were being studied. They were paid the going rate for physician record review. We met with each group of physicians (typically 4–8 for a hospital) to instruct them in the review process and make sure they understood the definitions. This was a crucial task, since "adverse event" was a new concept for many, and distinguishing treatment-caused injuries from complications of the disease was not something any had ever done.

We also made clear that the term "adverse event" did not mean there had been an error in care. They would find that some were caused by errors and others were not. Part of the purpose of the study was to find out how many there were of each. Despite this caution, we discovered later that many of them considered error the equivalent of negligence, that is, they resulted from the physician not being careful enough. In truth, at that time most of us more or less shared that point of view. The final design included a random sample of over 31,000 patients who were selected from 51 randomly selected acute care New York hospitals. Government hospitals and mental institutions were excluded. Study hospitals were asked to provide a list of all patients discharged in calendar year 1984.

But the surprising finding was that more than two-thirds of the injuries seemed to be potentially preventable. Reviewers were able to identify specific errors from information in the medical records for 58% of the AEs [4]; subsequent analysis revealed that an additional 11% of AEs resulted from failure to follow accepted practices, raising the total fraction of potentially preventable AEs to 69% [5]. Complications of the use of medications were the most common type.

We were very much aware of the limitations of our study—how far it could fall short of our goal of identifying every adverse event and only adverse events. The likelihood is that our numbers underestimated the number of AEs. There were opportunities at each stage for missing an adverse event. It is unlikely that we were overcounting. Reviewers would not "see" events that hadn't happened! On balance, we believed that our rates, shocking as they were, underestimated the true extent of harm. In fact, later studies would bear this out.

The implications of our findings were profound. If our rates were representative, i.e., if adverse event rates in hospitals across the country were similar to what we found in New York State, then nationwide 1.3 million patients were injured by medical care in American acute care hospitals that year, and 180,000 died from these injuries! These numbers were an order of magnitude higher than had ever been suggested. Medical injury was truly a hidden epidemic.

But I was struck with something else: more than two-thirds of the AE were caused by errors and systems failures that we could detect in the medical record. This meant that of the projected 180,000 deaths each year, more than 120,000 were potentially preventable. I was surprised that no one else in the study group found this particularly alarming or of interest. The focus of the study was on malpractice— the costs of injuries and who paid. But it was the fact that two-thirds were potentially preventable that captured my attention. Surely, we should be able to eliminate those—or at least some of them. Preventing these errors and failures could be a huge agenda for improvement. My colleagues disagreed and warned, "Don't go there. The doctors will hate you."

The results of the study were published in two papers in the New England Journal of Medicine in February 1991 [3, 4]. It got substantial local coverage in the New York media and some national notice. The New York State Medical Society was not pleased but made the best of it by claiming that the 1% negligence rate (27% of 3.7% injury rate) was quite low and showed that doctors were performing at a 99% perfect level! [6] But interest in the study faded quickly. No one knew what to do about it, so after a few commentaries from assorted parties, everyone, lay and professional, pretty much quit talking about it. The Medical Practice Study did one other thing: it determined the feasibility of no-fault insurance as an alternative to the tort system to compensate patients for medical injury. Malpractice suits only compensate patients whose injuries were caused by negligence and who succeed in winning a malpractice suit. Most people don't sue, and most of those who do don't win. The net result is that very few injured patients are compensated by the tort system. In a no-fault plan, all patients who suffer a treatment-caused injury are compensated for all its subsequent costs, irrespective of whether the injury was caused by error or negligence. Importantly, these costs also include lost wages, home care, and long-term disability care. To determine the feasibility of no-fault compensation, we did a follow-up study of the economic consequences of the adverse events. We interviewed the patients from our study who had been injured—or their next of kin if they had died—to determine the long-term effects of the injuries on the victims (such as permanent disability and inability to work), and we estimated their total costs, medical care, lost wages, disability.

Nonetheless, the Medical Practice Study had a profound impact. Although it was designed to address malpractice, its far greater significance came from the revelation of the horrendous extent of harm that resulted from routine medical care. Here for the first time was indisputable evidence that hundreds of thousands of people were being harmed every year by care intended to help them. And, for the first time, evidence that many of those injuries were potentially preventable. Patient safety was a much greater problem than any of us realized. But it would take some time for this to sink in for the medical profession and its leaders.

My critique: Twenty years after the Joint Commission, AOA, and one must presume, various state agencies, since each state licenses hospitals and doctors, had been seeking such information, and also seeking to respond to, and reduce such patient care tragedies; this intense study seems to have opened Pandora's box. Finally, in 1989 the results of a multi-year study revealed that thousands of patients have been *needlessly dying* in hospitals, and again, one must assume throughout the history of hospitals, and this revelation resulted in—The results of the study were published in two papers in the New England Journal of Medicine in February 1991 [3, 4]. It got substantial local coverage in the New York media and some national notice. But interest in the study faded quickly. Perhaps this is because we were fore warned; the AMA had always made clear that anything that might possibly make doctors look bad was unacceptable.

Plus, that last statement is not quite true. The results of that study had all the effect in Congress and all 50 state capitals as a tree falling in an empty forest, and the same disinterest, and selective stupidity has continued at every level of elected decision-making since.

Dr. Leape also misspoke; the efforts and results of that study were published in three articles in the New England Journal of Medicine. Part I and II were published in February 1991, and Part III published in July 1991, and I have copies of each article.

This multi-year study of *needless hospital deaths* was like the first shot in any war, and this war (an accurate word for what was to come) was and continues to be focused on how to begin to reduce such *needless* (there's that word again) tragedies that continue today, and with NO discernable reduction in carnage.

Becoming a patient in any hospital in America is like shooting craps in Las Vegas, not everyone will come out a winner.

Hospitals are no safer for patients today than they were in 1989 when the Brennan and Leape study was first reported, and there are clearly evident reasons why, but NO discernable interest in pursuing such evidence.

While the Brennan & Leape Report set the bar for future studies regarding needless hospital deaths, Congress was expanding the number of Federal Agencies tasked with helping make our Nation's hospitals safer. Agency for Healthcare Research & Quality (AHRQ), and National Practitioner Data Bank (NPDB) were created. AHRQ claims to be the lead Federal agency charged with improving the safety and quality of healthcare for all Americans. Over thirty years after their creation, and billions of dollars, and hospital safety is no better now than it was in 1989. Also, Congress allowed the AMA to so cripple the accountability mechanisms of the NPDB that it has been almost ineffective in its primary mission to provide effective accountability within hospital medical staffs. In essences, both agencies have proven to be monumental frauds.

It is difficult to attempt to describe the evolution of what was to become an enormous Quality of Care and Patient Safety army of experts centered around multiple Federal agencies (two more new agencies would be added to the mix in late 1990, and

2010) in a condensed manner worthy of understanding, but I will try by limiting this description to what I consider the more informative events, and the next BIG event was the IOM (now National Academy of Medicine) To Err Is Human report in 1999. Two selected quotes should be sufficient to illustrate what the army of experts have always touted as being a major accomplishment, while those two quotes demonstrate that report to be a meaningless deceit.

To Err Is Human, Building a Safer Health System, Institute of Medicine, November 1999

A variety of factors have contributed to the nation's epidemic of medical errors. One oft-cited problem arises from the decentralized and fragmented nature of the health care delivery system—or "nonsystematic" to some observers. Page 1

In this report, issued in September 1999, the committee lays out a comprehensive strategy by which government, health care providers, industry, and consumers can reduce preventable medical errors. Concluding that the know-how already exists to prevent many of these mistakes, the report sets as a minimum goal a 50 percent reduction in errors over the next five years.

My critique: Everything they were doing should have been stopped the moment "some observers" considered the System to be a non-system! The current System is now and has always been devoid of any true systematic characteristics, and that fact is one of the most fundamental reasons why the current System is far less effective in-patient safety than it should or could be. And that statement on Page 2; "the report sets as a minimum goal a 50 percent reduction in errors over the next five years" clearly demonstrates the entire report to be a colossal, bureaucratic lie perpetrated on the unknowing public. But Dr. Leape's book clearly illustrates just how great that bureaucratic life is and continues to be.

Two important events were taking place within this army of experts, Congress was adding a 4th Federal agency, National Quality Forum (NQF) just as the IOM was releasing To Err Is Human, and the following exchange took place. John Eisenberg, Director of AHRQ was asked to brief President Clinton on the report and found that Clinton had not only read the entire report but understood it. He asked John whether it was possible, as the IOM report challenged, for healthcare to reduce preventable deaths by 50% in 5 years. John said yes, or even in 2 years or 1 year—because hospitals would manipulate their measures to make it appear that happened.

So, John said yes, or even in 2 years or 1 year—because hospitals would manipulate their measures to make it appear that happened. WOW! That statement should tell you all one needs to know about To Err Is Human, and the veracity of that army of Quality of Care and Patient Safety experts; *hospitals would manipulate their measures,* and *AMA does not tolerate negative comments about doctors.* So let me summarize the truth about all the efforts of that army of experts for over 3 decades prior to COVID.

Needless Hospital Deaths Track Record

1990 Brennan, Leape, et al: The seminal estimate of 98,000 NHDs annually after four years of research in up-state New York hospitals. Brennan made the first report in 1989.

2000 IOM To Err Is Human: Used the Brennan & Leape estimate of 98,000 as their benchmark. Dr. Leape actively participated as a member of one of the two committees.

2009 Dead By Mistake, Hearst Newspapers: "but all available research indicates that the death toll from preventable medical injuries approaches 200,000 per year in the U.S.

2013 John James, PhD, Journal of Patient Safety, September: Estimated NHDs at more than 400,000 per year, and serious harm seems to be 10-20-fold more common than lethal harm.

2013 ProPublica, September: Drs. Leape, Makary, and Classen soundly support James' findings. Dr. Leape was proclaimed the Father of Patient Safety in BMJ Careers in Dec. 2012.

2016 Dr. Marty Makary suggested that medical errors are the third leading cause of deaths behind heart disease and cancer.

Dr. Leape ends his book at 2015, and one assumes his active participation in all the future efforts by that army of experts so there is no mention of Dr. Makary's claim that medical errors are the 3rd leading cause of deaths in the U.S. 27 years after Brennan & Leape set the initial bar for *needless hospital deaths*.

Everything about that army of experts that has been centered around those 5 Federal agencies tasked with making hospital care far safer for patients, while they were accepting the fact that hospitals would be manipulating their measures. Doctors are the key to all medical care, and the AMA has long been the straw that stirs the Medical Profession's drink in American, and the AMA contributions to the efforts to make our hospitals far safer is next.

American Medical Association

I have written four books, and a 2nd edition on my 3rd book about the Healthcare Delivery System (HCDS) (doctors, hospitals and surgery centers) and the pervious chapters here make it clear that I have been challenging that "System" from inside that "System" for over 40 years. Still, today, Quality of Care and Patient Safety Experts are in strong agreement, that System is "broken" (a very poor word for such a critical understanding, yet it gives an accurate assessment).

The Healthcare Delivery System is enormous, and complex therefore one book can hardly cover that system's current shortcomings, and the same can be said for both the AMA, and the Joint Commission. Therefore, I am left with only my ability to share some of my views about those two major components of the HCDS, and some examples of how each of those components have contributed to the current, highly flawed status of that system.

There is an estimated 800-850,000 MD and DO (osteopaths) doctors practicing medicine in America today, and the vast majority of them are doing just that, practicing their personal specialty of medicine. Most doctors are not members of the AMA and its 3-levels of membership, national, state, and local.

Also, most doctors currently practicing medicine are *average at best*. Every medical school graduating class is made up by three distinct groups; the cream, middle, and lower (those who were successful in meeting sufficient graded standards, but not by a wide margin). And those three groups will vary in each graduating class, with some classes having a large segment of the cream, and vice versa. So, basically, most practicing doctors are average, and that should be as expected. I have survived 5 surgeries, 3 major, and 2 gastrointestinal scopings, and I assume not all of those doctors were necessarily in the cream of their graduating class, yet my advanced age provides credit to each doctor's capability.

Those doctors who seek leadership positions in hospitals, AMA levels of service, and various levels of professional decision-making are the ones who continue to perpetuate the unprofessional and unethical aspects of their profession, i.e., Code of Silence, and the curse of medical malpractice litigation, and a visit behind the AMA curtain should well illustrate this perspective of Organized Medicine. But it all begins with medical malpractice.

Medical Malpractice

What is it & Who decides?

First, I despise the term, *medical malpractice*. All doctors are humans, and all humans make mistakes, therefore, even the best doctors make mistakes, and not all medical complications are negligent care. Therefore, I prefer the term *questionable patient care*.

Questionable Patient Care (is it or isn't it) is, in my opinion, a far better term for two reasons; "medical malpractice" is a pejorative that instantly labels an unknown as an accepted negative and because not all medical complications are due to substandard care. I would always support a doctor in the review of a case where all reasonable patient care had been provided as I would the patient in cases where substandard care was clear.

Malpractice: Professional misconduct or failure to properly discharge professional duties by failing to meet the standard of care required of a professional: Legal Medicine 5th edition, American College of Legal Medicine. Unfortunately, the American College of Legal Medicine failed to clarify who determines what the "standard of care" is, but an AMA President-Elect would clarify that issue.

2003 Donald J. Palmisano, MD, JD, AMA President-Elect filmed a video in the AMA Washington DC office entitled *Understanding the Medical Malpractice Crisis*, and very early in that video Dr. Palmisano said.

"Doctors, under the law, if you're treating a patient and you fall below a standard of care SET BY THE LAW and those standards are determined by EXPERTS, and that directly causes damage to the patient, that's medical malpractice."
(Emphasis added).

I discovered that video in the medical library at Greenville Memorial Hospital while doing research for my first book, *First Do No Harm, The Cure for Medical Malpractice*, and I still have my copy that I obtained upon request from the AMA.

My first reaction upon watching that video was, "My God, they have fallen on their own sword." With time, I came to realize that that definition of medical malpractice documents our Nation's Medical Profession's total abdication of their professional responsibility to attempt to provide any effective means of professional peer review for instances of questionable patient care. Other quotes by Dr. Palmisano are also revealing.

Need for an expert: *"To determine the standard of care; to determine the height of the "low hurdles" in the review of patient care."*

"The law requires a MINIMALLY Acceptable Level of Care, thus my analogy to the "low hurdle". Source: A Primer of Malpractice Law—Intrepid Resources (owned by Dr. Palmisano) June 28, 2002. St. Mary's Hospital Medical Staff peer review process for Agnes certainly determined a very low hurdle for her 4 months of treatment.

"We do know that the liability system does not measure negligence."

Source: Newshour, PBS, Jan. 16, 2003, Subject: Medical Malpractice.

Ray Suarez apparently failed to ask Dr. Palmisano, "Who does measure medical negligence?" Sadly, medical negligence is rarely 'measured' by anyone.

A special note: Dr. Palmisano sadly suffered a fatal accident in his home in late November 2022, and reading his obituary recounts a person with over-whelming attributes, but there is naturally no mention of some of his greatest, and most harmful to the public contributions to the Dark Side of the AMA and his Medical Profession. Dr. Palmisano was the principal architect of the AMA Litigation Center, and my exposure of that enemy of every patient who may have been harmed by negligent medical care follows.

And the AMA contribution at the same time (2003) widely circulated a brochure in doctors' offices:

AMA Brochure—Will Your Doctor Be There? 2003

"The PRIMARY cause of America's medical liability crisis is Overzealous Personal Injury Attorneys who put their pocketbooks before patients."

How do attorneys become the "primary cause" of our Nation's 4-decade old medical malpractice crisis? *The primary cause* is a very important *label* in the practice of medicine. I performed 35 autopsies during my six-month rotation on Pathology during my second year of my three-year oral surgery residency. The *primary purpose* of an autopsy is to identify the *primary,* and then also the *secondary causes,* of the death of that deceased patient. Doctors stopped doing autopsies because they were demonstrating too many inaccurate and poor diagnostic mistakes.

Dr. Palmisano had also said, "What we need are more debates regarding medical malpractice", and I took him at his word. I received the first copies of *First Do No Harm* in March 2004, and I flew to Chicago in June, and attended the AMA Annual Meeting, surreptitiously for a couple of days until finally I had an opportunity to approach Dr. Palmisano as if he was alone.

Dr. Palmisano, I am Dr. Ira Williams, and I recently published a book entitled *First Do No Harm, The Cure for Medical Malpractice.* You said that what was needed was more debates about that subject, and I have come here to offer myself for such a debate.

Dr. Williams, I am much too busy to consider your offer currently. And with that he walked away. Although he was, on that day becoming AMA Past-President, Dr. Palmisano would prove to be very busy, and not in a way beneficial to the public, but more on that later.

Dr. Palmisano became AMA President in June 2003, and in a two-year period, if one connects the dots, the following event and declarations took place:

- Litigation Center came alive in North Carolina.
- Malpractice is harmful patient care beneath a standard of care *set by the law.*
- The liability system *does not measure negligence.*
- Law *requires a minimally acceptable level of care.*
- The Malpractice Crisis was (is) *caused by overzealous attorneys.*

What is too easily missed in all of the above? AMA and their constituent state and local societies are like the American Hospital Association and its constituent state societies, all *associations* are membership organizations, and therefore devoid of authority over their respective members. North Carolina Medical Board, an agency created by the highest power of that state and given regulatory authority was necessary to do the AMA–State Medical Societies bidding. No authority equals No regulatory ability, and that equals No accountability, even when that accountability appears perhaps to have been misdirected.

Medical malpractice facts never mentioned:

There is NO malpractice without expert witness testimony. Except in cases of res ipsa loquitur (the thing speaks for itself)

Res ipsa loquitur medical malpractice cases are extremely rare, i.e., a doctor amputates the wrong arm or leg, the thing speaks for itself). Civil court judges determine its use, or non-use, and are very reluctant to apply it. I served as the second surgeon in three separate cases in Madison, and I felt that each of those 3 cases were worthy of being considered res ipsa loquitur due to the gross negligence by the first surgeon in each case. But no judge in Wisconsin would have ever even considered such a ruling. But, back to; there is no malpractice without expert witness testimony. Therefore, the goal of the AMA has always been to do everything possible to make becoming an expert witness for the Plaintiff (patient) a very dangerous undertaking.

1997 – Testifying is practicing medicine:

AMA policy says that when a physician gives medical legal testimony, it's considered the practice of medicine and it should be subject to peer review. The Association's House of Delegates passed the resolution in 1997 and reaffirmed it in 1998, 1999 and 2000.

1999 – Litigation Center of the AMA-State Medical Societies:

Mission Statement: The mission of the Litigation Center is to be an effective legal advocate in representing the interests of the medical profession in the courts by bringing cases of broad impact and by serving as an information and advocacy clearinghouse for medical societies and related groups. The Litigation Center will perform its mission in accordance with the policies of the AMA.

These bylaws set forth the rules and procedures under which the Litigation Center will operate. And by 2003, the very state medical society had created a Litigation Center component, and Dr. Palmisano had had a leading position in this new AMA initiative.

Dr. Palmisano, MD, JD, as AMA Past-President was the AMA Board Representative on the Litigation Center Executive Committee during its creation and in 2002 when Mr. Keene, NCMS General Counsel and Dr. Jaufmann's paths conveniently crossed those individuals would see an opportunity that would allowed the North Carolina Medical Society and Medical Examining Board to lead the nation in rooting out nefarious expert witnesses for patients who may have died due to questionable circumstances.

North Carolina Medical Society, and North Carolina Medical Board would combine their efforts to initiate the first active implementation of their state's Litigation Center, and it would not be pretty because it would begin with the needless death of a young man who was merely seeking to have a medical periodically necessary procedure to be repeated.

But to understand this story it must begin at the beginning, with the birth of a son, but not the completely happy birth every parent dream of. This son began life with a life-changing impediment. My wife and I had two sons, and I know the joy of the birth of one to "carry the name forward'. But these parents were denied such complete joy, and unknowingly, they were to experience one of life's greatest tragedies, the early loss of that son.

A chronological path of parallel events, one involving a highly questionable hospital death and the other involving the highest level of leaders within the AMA and every state's medical society, must be followed in order to take a reader behind the curtain of how Organized Medicine seeks to deny the public legal justice. Hopefully, most readers will try to picture their reaction if a similar set of circumstances occurred in their life. For others, the events described here will become all-too real.

First Event

1975: A young North Carolina couple celebrates the joy of the birth of a son. Unfortunately, their initial joy was tempered when their infant was diagnosed with congenital hydrocephalus, the swelling of the brain due to excess buildup of cerebral spinal fluid. There are certain factors regarding cerebral hydrocephalus that must be understood before proceeding with the important aspects of this first event, but without going into great detail regarding all of the medical factors associated with that congenital abnormality. I leave the reader with my source, Google.

Congenital hydrocephalus requires a neurosurgeon to insert a cerebral shunt, or drain, between the brain cavity and other anatomical cavities within the patient's body in order to redirect the excessive cerebral spinal fluid. Once the initial cerebral shunt, or drain, is placed, it will need, like most drains typically do, to be replaced periodically. Furthermore, this type of surgical procedure, like all other surgical procedures, is susceptible to a number of complications associated with shunt placement. The common symptoms often resemble the new onset of hydrocephalus such as headaches, nausea, vomiting, double vision, and an alteration of consciousness. Furthermore, the shunt failure rate two years after pump and implantation has been estimated to be as high as 50%.

Note: *Cerebral shunts require periodic replacement, those procedures have a clearly understood list of possible postoperative complications, even possibly leading to death, but many people can live healthy lives IF provided with adequate medical care. Each of those points plays an important part in this First Event.*

1995: Bill, the central figure in this First Event, had successfully dealt with his congenital abnormality for 20 years, including periodic shunt replacement procedures, sufficiently to allow him to leave home and attend an in-state university. During his academic year Bill faced the need for another periodic shunt replacement procedure. Bill consulted with Dr. Victor Karanen and a drain replacement procedure was agreed upon and scheduled. Bill was also told, and accepted, that following that procedure Bill's postoperative care would be the responsibility of the surgeon on call, Neurosurgeon #2.

That surgery appeared to go well, but about four hours later, and after Dr. Bruce Jaufmann had assumed responsibility for Dr. Karanen's patients, Bill got a headache and grew agitated. There appeared to be some indication that the nursing staff called Dr. Jaufmann to report Bill's complaint of increasing *headache,* and Dr.

Jaufmann did not immediately respond by coming to see his new medical responsibility.

The rest of Bill's unfortunate story can be summarized with these few details; by the time Dr. Jaufmann arrived at Bill's bedside <u>his</u> <u>patient</u> was in critical condition, including heart stoppage. Bill was revived, and Dr. Jaufmann performed an emergency brain operation, but that surgery proved to be too late. Bill was put on an artificial respirator and died 18 days later. Bill's parents were left to grieve the, perhaps needless, but certainly highly questionable loss of their son, and also left with *Sue or Forget It*.

Note: *Most of the information contained above has been taken from an article in the Raleigh News & Observer, Sunday, September 1, 2002, and written by Sarah Avery and Matthew Eisley. I have quoted multiple portions of that article and will again later.*

Sue or Forget It

Throughout the history of health care in America the Public has overwhelmingly been left with medical malpractice litigation (Sue or Forget It) as the primary source for the review of questionable patient care. Bill's parents found themselves on the horns of that dilemma while trying to cope with having to bury their young son and wondering what happened. Bill's parents decided they must enter that strange and adversarial land of medical malpractice litigation, where each side is determined to "take no prisoners!" I know of what I say regarding medical malpractice litigation.

What do people need to know if and when they feel they must sue a doctor?

First, they must understand that they must deal with:

- Psychological burden of instantly becoming a *pariah* within their medical community because there will be definite repercussions.
- Endurance, because malpractice litigation typically requires three or more years, and the stigma is constant.
- Financial burden, even on a contingency basis. I never served as an expert witness for financially

sound plaintiffs, but I only served as an expert witness for plaintiffs who deserved their day in court.

Second, absolutes they need to initiate the litigation process:

- Attorney, qualified in medical malpractice litigation. I had the misfortune of being involved in a malpractice trial with a good attorney, but unfortunately, lacking in medical malpractice litigation experience. That trial did not go well.
- Qualified expert witness (a vanishing breed) because *there is NO medical malpractice without expert witness testimony*! That *fact* plays a very important point in this entire chapter.
- Res ipsa loquitur (Latin: the thing speaks for itself). No expert witness is required IF they amputate the wrong limb, etc. This exception is a malpractice litigation rarity, requested more often by plaintiff's attorneys than allowed by trial judges.

The Die is Cast

1997: Bill's parents made the determination that they needed to enter the medical malpractice litigation arena, and they were able to fulfill the first requirement, they obtained qualified medical malpractice attorneys. Those attorneys were then able to acquire the services of a Florida-based neurosurgeon, experienced as an expert witness in such cases, and who just happened to have a North Carolina medical license, not that that was necessary, but that fact becomes most important to the rest of this story.

Note: *I obtained a Wisconsin license to practice oral surgery at the completion of my three-year residency in Milwaukee that allowed me to practice oral surgery in Madison, Wisconsin. I also possessed a license to practice in Tennessee, my home state, obtained in 1961 and another license to practice in Louisiana obtained in the summer of 1962 during my internship. I retained both as active licenses for many years.*

Medical malpractice litigation process requires several preliminary steps:

- Qualified attorney to obtain all medical records, review those records and accept the plaintiffs as clients, and obtain an expert witness to do the same.
- Expert witness must review the records, determine if he or she is qualified to testify and if the records support an expert witness opinion that the patient care did not meet a reasonable standard of care, then accept the responsibility as an expert witness in that case.
- The judge must determine that all necessary requirements have been satisfied in order to set the case for trial. Some states require the expert witness(es) to first certify in writing the factors upon which they will base their testimony of substandard care. I have provided several such letters for judicial acceptance and was never turned down.
- Discovery process begins following judicial approval of the plaintiff's case. Depositions of defendant doctors, plaintiffs, expert witnesses, and any other persons, as determined by the trial judge, are taken. Expert witness depositions are taken under oath, reviewed by the person deposed in order to make corrections, if necessary, and accepted as equal to sworn testimony given in a trial.

1997: Dr. Gary Lustgarten provided his deposition in the plaintiff's (Bill's parents) malpractice cases against Drs. Keranen and Jaufmann and the hospital for the negligent death of their son. Dr. Karanen and the hospital settled their cases with the plaintiffs shortly after they had obtained and read the Expert Witness' deposition.

Note: *I have given about 40 malpractice depositions in surgical malpractice cases involving both physicians and oral surgeons, and far more of those cases settled after my deposition than later went to trial.*

But a very important series of events took place in this particular malpractice litigation case and each of those events must be noted and connected.

Dr. Jaufmann, the surgeon on call who had presumably accepted responsibility for Bill's postoperative care, and who failed to examine Bill in response to the first sign of postoperative complication, refused to settle his case. Some medical malpractice insurance policies are written in a manner that leaves the doctor in control of any determination of settling prior to trial and other such policies permit the insurance company to make that determination.

Two separate events coincidentally came together that enabled the AMA to clearly demonstrate who comes first in their professional obligations: doctors or patients, and their grieving loved ones.

First Event: Bill's parents, for reasons of their own, but understandable reasons to me, elected not to pursue further litigation efforts that would require them to relive Bill's questionable death in a trial months away, and before a jury of people with no medical expertise. Therefore, the only questions ever asked and answered regarding the circumstances of Bill's untimely death were contained in that Expert Witness' deposition, and they were presumably asked and answered. AMA and the North Carolina Medical Society would decide five years later that the malpractice litigation review (Sue or Forget It) of Bill's highly questionable death did not meet 'their standards of medical review",

Second Event: Also in 1997: AMA began formulating a process to unite themselves with all 50 state medical societies in the creation of what became the **Litigation Center** about the same time as Bill's highly questionable death and malpractice litigation process was seemingly coming to a close. And Bill's death and malpractice litigation process would become the centerpiece used to christen that new AMA-State Medical Societies creation to protect doctors from *evil plaintiff's expert witnesses*, who just happen to be an absolute necessity in almost every medical malpractice civil trial ever conducted in our courts for over 150 years.

AMA Process Begins in 1997
amednews.com April 8, 2002

The Newspaper for America's Physicians
On the hot seat: Physician expert witnesses:

With scrutiny high and the other side out to get the "hired gun", court appearances can be a trial for physicians who serve as expert witnesses.

1997: Bill's parents accepted the settlement with Dr. Karanen and the hospital and decided not to further pursue litigation against Dr. Jaufmann even thought that is the surgeon on call who failed to respond immediately to Bill's clinical sign of possible post-operative complication. Simultaneously, AMA House of Delegates was laying the groundwork for future assaults on patient's expert witnesses, as we shall see.

Regardless of what some might say, I believe too much cannot be made of this **Second Event** and the event to follow. But first, there are several considerations one should be aware of regarding the AMA, and all associations.

Associations are *membership organizations*, and as such, they have NO authority over their members. Any threat of possible conduct review by an association would be met with, "I just resigned my membership." Yet federal and state decision makers have always accepted medical and hospital associations as though they possessed such authority over their members. AMA is estimated to have less than 30% of the nation's doctors as members, yet their House of Delegates were presuming they were sufficiently powerful to suddenly (over four years) make new expert witness law, and have that new law accepted throughout Organized Medicine. And folks they did it and got away with it. Now I will show you how they got away with it.

Litigation Center of the AMA-State Medical Societies

AMA began creating the Litigation Center and recruiting state medical societies to join them in the late 90s and was successful in having all 50 state medical societies as active members by 2003. But this tale of two simultaneous events involving the questionable death of Bill in 1995 and the assumed closing of his parent's litigation process in 1997 was to gain new life thanks to the AMA-State Medical Societies Litigation Center.

The Litigation Center's Executive Committee contained 11 members, and 9 of those members represented 8 state medical societies and the District of Columbia in 2002. But one Executive Committee member stands out from all of the rest regarding Bill's questionable death seven years earlier.

Stephen W. Keene was in 2002 (and continues to be) North Carolina Medical Society General Counsel & Deputy Executive Vice President, Government Affairs & Health Policy.

Second Event Begins–But how?

Who called whom first? Did Dr. Jaufmann, still burning with indignation five years after Bill's parents had ended their quest for medical justice, somehow heard about this relatively new AMA-State Medical Society Litigation Center for the *peer review* of expert witness testimony? OR did NCMS General Counsel Stephen Keene recognize an opportunity to test this new professional device for reviewing any plaintiff's (patient's) expert witness' testimony? As an experienced plaintiff's expert witness in numerous malpractice cases across the nation I know what I believe about who called whom first, but I will leave it to others to decide. After being called a "hired gun" by every defense attorney I ever faced I understand all too well the medical profession's mind-set regarding malpractice litigation. But fortunately, we have additional information to help in making such a judgment.

Note: *Back to the Raleigh News & Observer, Sunday, September 1, 2002, article written by Sarah Avery and Matthew Eisley. Here they will describe the AMA-State Medical Societies Litigation Center in action, while ably assisted by the North Carolina Medical Board, to produce a perfect storm of medical profession pursuit for practitioner integrity and ethical conduct. All information taken from that article is quoted as written, except for the deletion of names and selected (Emphasis added).*

Raleigh News & Observer
Surgeon Fights for N.C. License

In the 20 years that Dr. Lustgarten has testified as an expert witness in medical malpractice lawsuits, he has always been prepared to defend his position against an equally qualified authority on the opposing side. Never did he anticipate he would have to defend his license to practice medicine because of what he had said in court.

But the North Carolina Medical Board Stripped Dr. Lustgarten of his North Carolina practicing privileges in July 2002 because of his testimony in 1997, and that decision is raising questions about how medical malpractice is controlled in North Carolina.

At issue is the North Carolina board's legal authority to make such a ruling. The board said Dr. Lustgarten was either dishonest or incompetent when he testified that the care two previous surgeons provided led to the death of a patient (Even though the hospital and Dr. Karanen settled the 1997 case prior to its going to trial—my thought).

The board's action may be the first case of its kind in the nation, although the Federation of State Medical Boards does not keep track. It's the first such case in North Carolina. (Emphasis added) [**Note:** I know of one other similar case that involved a case in Florida and an expert witness in California that took place during the same time-frame, but slightly later.]

"We need expert witnesses who will testify truthfully and fairly," a lawyer for the North Carolina Medical Board said during Dr. Lustgarten's July hearing. " If we permit our licensees to give testimony that clearly misstates the standard of care in North Carolina, then we're going to corrupt the system we have. We cannot permit it." That North Carolina board attorney went on to say that "Dr. Lustgarten's' testimony was outrageous."

But Dr. Jaufmann did not drop the matter, maintaining that Dr. Laustgarten had slandered his reputation. He filed a complaint with the state medical board. "This is not a difference of opinion." Dr. Jaufmann said in an interview. "There are certain acceptable standards and certain truths in neurosurgery." "Simply put," Dr. Jaufmann said, "Dr. Lustgarten lied."

In addition to policing its ranks for doctors who are felons, frauds, drunks, drug addicts or otherwise incompetent, the 12-member medical board can punish members for conduct that is "contrary to honesty, justice or good morals." That's the provision the board cited when, in April, it agreed with Dr. Jaufmann's assertion that Dr. Lustgarten knew or should have known that the doctors and nurses tending Bill did not violate any standards of care. The board summoned Dr. Lustgarten to a hearing in July.

In a five-page response, Dr. Lustgarten countered that he had merely voiced his opinion. He also pointed out that his North Carolina license, which he had received in 1981 when he briefly considered setting up a practice here, was inactive. And he asked the board to delay its hearing because he was required to appear in another legal case.

The board declined to postpone the hearing and rejected Dr. Lustgarten's subsequent request to testify over the phone in a conference call. Dr. Lustgarten failed to hire an attorney to appear on his behalf, so he offered no defense.

Testifying for the board were Dr. Jaufmann and an attorney hired by Dr. Jaufmann and his insurance company for Bill's parents' 1997 lawsuit. That attorney told the board that Dr. Lustgarten's testimony underpinned a questionable claim – even though that attorney had agreed to settle the claim for Dr. Karanen when that surgeon and the hospital settled prior to trial in1997.

"It allowed a case to spend two years in litigation that shouldn't have been there", that attorney told the medical board. "Dr. Jaufmann refused to settle the case because he had been called a liar, which stood to hurt his reputation. Dr. Jaufmann was extremely upset."

The board voted unanimously after 20 minutes of deliberation to revoke Dr. Luatgarten's *North Carolina license.* (Emphasis added)

The 2002 president of the American Medical Association said he welcomes the kind of oversight in the North Carolina Medical Board offered. He said many malpractice lawsuits are justified, as are the jury awards. Other times, however, unworthy cases are made to seem legitimate when so-called experts testify falsely, he said.

A personal injury attorney and lecturer at the Duke University School of Law said the current system already discourages many legitimate cases from being filed, because it takes time and money to find a doctor willing to appear as an expert witness. The medical board's action against Dr. Lustgarten, legal experts said, would serve to scare the few doctors willing to take the stand.

The Executive Vice President and Chief Executive Officer of the Federation of State Medical Boards said he anticipates no such backlash. "Physicians have a societal obligation to protect the public, and I believe physicians will heed that call and testify when cases warrant." *"What may happen,"* he said, *"is that more boards will follow North Carolina's lead."* (Emphasis added)

For Dr. Lustgarten, the issue is both professional and personal. He could face a similar revocation of his license in Florida, effectively ending his medical career. His testimony in Bill's case has already resulted in a six- month suspension by the American Association of Neurological Surgeons.

The North Carolina Medical Board president, a professor of surgery and biochemistry at the Brody School of Medicine at East Carolina University, told Dr. Jaufmann,*" this will send a big message."* (Emphasis added) But, that message would not stand the test of time.

Dr. Lustgarten appealed the Board's ruling and the order to revoke his North Carolina medical license (which also threatened the status of his Florida license and his professional future) in April 2003 and the Board's decision to revoke his license was vacated and replaced with a one-year suspension in 2004. Dr. Lusgarten was still not done.

Dr. Lustgarten appealed that appellate decision in 2004, and the next appellate decision by the same judge made no change in his previous decision. Dr. Lustgarten appealed that decision in 2005, and the true facts of this entire matter finally were exposed.

North Carolina Court of Appeals
Filed: 6 June 2006

Dr. Jaufmann had recorded in the patient's record that the patient's cerebral spinal fluid was *not under increased pressure at the time of his second surgery* However the patient did not respond to that second surgery and subsequently died.

Dr. Lustgarten was accused by defense attorneys using his deposition testimony during the trial that he had accused Dr. Jaufmann of falsifying medical records. Dr. Lustgarten denied ever claiming such an accusation. However, Dr. Lustgarten had testified that there were four clinically evident reasons for his conclusion that the patient's cerebral spinal fluid pressure had to be elevated. Therefore Dr. Lustgarten had difficulty believing Dr. Jaufmann's notation to the contrary.

It was further pointed out that there were at least three highly qualified healthcare professionals in close proximity to the patient when Dr. Jaufmann removed the original drain that had been placed by Dr. Karanen. An anesthesiologist, a surgical (scrub) nurse and a circulating nurse were present at that moment and yet in testimony it was stated that nobody else who witnessed the removal of that drain "recalls whether spinal fluid spurted out or not." Basically, the only one who commented on that was Dr. Jaufmann, and the others participating in that surgical procedure "saw no evil, heard no evil, and certainly, spoke no evil."

The North Carolina Medical Board is statutorily imbued with the authority to regulate the practice of medicine and surgery for the benefit and protection of the people of North Carolina. The Board has the power to deny, annul, suspend, or revoke the license of a license holder found by the Board to have committed unprofessional conduct. AS such the Board is an occupational licensing agency, which is governed by Article 3A of the North Carolina Administrative Procedure Act. Occupational licensing agency means any board which is established for the primary purpose with a particular profession, and which is authorized to issue and revoke licenses.

North Carolina Medical Board, in revoking Dr. Lustgarten's license based that action upon multiple reasons to support their contention that Dr. Lustgarten had absolutely no direct evidence to support his extremely serious accusation.

The Superior Court ruled that his finding was supported by substantial evidence in the record including the four clinically evident reasons Dr. Lustgarten stated. These observations provided a good faith evidentiary basis for Dr. Lustgarten's opinion that Dr. Jaufmann notation WAS NOT CREDIBLE. Furthermore, the record is clear that Dr. Lustgarten was content to state no more than his opinion that Dr. Jaufmann's note in the patient's record was faulty.

Superior Court three-judge appellate panel found no evidence in the record to support the Medical Board's decision to revoke Dr. Lustgarten's license. Therefore, the Board erred by finding that Dr. Lustgarten leveled a groundless accusation and that the previous Superior court appeals processes had erroneously applied the whole record test to affirm the Medical Board's determination. Therefore, the Superior Court's previous orders affirming the Board's decision were reversed and the disciplinary proceedings against Dr. Lustgarten were dismissed. The Court's final order reversed and remanded by unanimous consent of the three judges in June 2006.

North Carolina Medical Board's executive director was quoted in a state newspaper the day after the North Carolina Court of Appeals had revoked that Board's previous finding in 2002. "The Medical Board's position was and probably still is that Dr. Lustgarten's testimony in that case was at best reckless." I like to think of it as, the NCMB, and the NCMS had been "taken to the woodshed" by the NC Court of Appeals, and their pride had been hurt, for good reason.

Eleven years of professional tragedy compounded by professional malfeasance and every state medical society still has a Litigation Center component, so I will provide some additional summation to compare in the NCMB executive director's unqualified estimation of neurosurgical testimony.

Questions Never Asked

Where was the North Carolina Medical Board, with their profound expertise regarding neurosurgical standards of care, in 1995 when young, otherwise healthy, Bill died under highly questionable immediate post-operative circumstances?

Why did the North Carolina Medical Board not provide examples from Dr. Lustgarten's deposition of clear evidence of how "he lied under oath"? I still have copies of "lies under oath" given in a deposition by a Defense Expert Witness who just happened to be the Chairman of a Surgery Department at the local medical school and teaching hospital. I wager the AMA-Medical Societies Litigation Center has never collaborated with a state medical examining board to review the sworn testimony of an expert witness who happened to be testifying in defense of the accused practitioner, but more on this later.

These parallel events involving Bill's unfortunate death and the emergence of the new and dynamic AMA-State Medical Societies Litigation Center, aided by very willing state medical examining boards, raises far more questions, and provides far fewer answers than the involved components of Organized Medicine would wish to be forced to confront. But I will raise some of those questions here and provide some of my highly opinionated responses. I also said that I would name names (when necessary) and give dates, because it is impossible to create a well-defined picture of a complex issue unless one "connects the dots" with names and dates. So, let's begin with:

Evolution of the Medical Malpractice Dilemma

Our nation's Medical Profession's Leadership took the easy way out and therefore they have always left the Public with Sue or Forget It! Doctors don't know how to fairly judge another doctor's questionable patient care and they have never known or ever attempted to try to learn how.

Organized Medicine
One of its finest hours

Organized Medicine was represented solely by the founding of the American Medical Association (AMA) in 1847, followed by the American College of Surgeons (ACS) in 1913 and the American College of Physicians (ACP) in 1915. Paul Starr best described the true measure of how doctors dominated health care in America throughout most of its history in his Pulitzer Prize winning book, The Social Transformation of American Medicine (1982). I quote:

"Yet the replacement of a competitive orientation with a corporate consciousness required more than common interests. It required a transfer of power to the group, and this was what began to happen in medicine around 1900 with changes in its social structure. Physicians came increasingly to rely on each other's goodwill for their access to patients and facilities. Physicians also depended more on their colleagues for defense against malpractice suits, which were increasing in frequency. The courts, in working out the rules of liability for medical practice in the late nineteenth century, had set as the standard of care that of the local community where the physicians practiced. This limited possible expert testimony against physicians to their immediate colleagues. By adopting the "locality rule", the courts prepared the way for granting considerable power to the local medical society, for it became almost impossible for patients to get testimony against a physician who was a member. Medical societies began to make malpractice defense a direct service. Shortly after the turn of the century, doctors in New York, Chicago, and Cleveland organized common defense funds. The Massachusetts Medical Society began handling malpractice suits in 1908. During the next ten years, it supported accused physicians in all but three of the ninety-four cases it received. Only twelve of these ninety-one cases went to trial, all save one resulting in a victory for the doctor. For its first twenty years, the defense fund of the medical society of the state of Washington won every case it fought. Because of their ability to protect their members, medical societies were able to get low insurance rates, while doctors who did not belong could scarcely get any insurance protection. This provided the sort of "selected incentive" that medical societies needed to help them attract members. Professional ostracism carried increasingly serious consequences: denial of hospital privileges, loss of referrals, loss of malpractice insurance, and in extreme cases, loss of a license to practice. The local medical fraternity became the arbiter of a doctor's position and fortune, and he could no longer choose to ignore it. By making the county societies the gatekeeper to membership in any higher professional group, the AMA had recognized and strengthened the position of the local fraternity, as well as bolstering its own organizational underpinnings."

I considered Professor Starr's description of how the AMA controlled the practice of medicine in America 100 years ago similar to the way Al Capone controlled Chicago, the home of the AMA Headquarters, for several years, though out-right terror.

A Department Head at the Arnold School of Public Health at the University of South Carolina in Columbia SC told me that Professor Starr's book is still required reading at their institution more than thirty years after it was published. Both AMA and Arnold School of Public Health reinforce the understanding that old habits are hard to change.

Those who cannot remember the past are condemned to repeat it.

—George Santayana

State Medical Examining Boards

Federation of State Medical Boards:
About State Medical Boards:

Medicine is a regulated profession because of the potential harm to the public if an incompetent or impaired physician is licensed to practice. To protect the public from the unprofessional, improper, unlawful, fraudulent and/or income incompetent practice of medicine, each of the fifty states, the District of Columbia, and the U.S. territories has a medical practice act that defines the practice of medicine and *delegates* the *authority* to *enforce the law* to a state medical board.

State medical boards licensed physicians, investigate complaints, discipline those who violate the law, conduct position evaluations, and facilitate rehabilitation of physicians where appropriate. By following up on complaints, medical boards give the public a way to enforce basic standards of competence and ethical behavior in their physicians, and physicians a way to protect the integrity of their profession. State medical boards also adopt policies and guidelines related to the practice of medicine. There are currently 70 state medical boards authorized to regulate allopathic and osteopathic physicians.

The 10th amendment of the United States Constitution authorizes states to establish laws and regulations protecting the health, safety, and general welfare of their citizens. In response to the 10th amendment, each state legislature enacted a Medical Practice Act that defines the proper practice of medicine and responsibility of the medical board to regulate that practice (all italics above are emphasis added).

Response: Every state's medical examining board is currently over 100 years old and those three paragraphs above this response may describe the theoretical purpose of such state created regulatory agencies, but those paragraphs do not describe the reality of how any of those state boards have performed in their attempt to satisfy their original mandate. Try to find even one state medical examining board that can provide clear evidence of even coming close to achieving their original mandate.

The AMA-State Medical Societies Litigation Center and the North Carolina Medical Society – North Carolina Medical Board collaboration in 2002 provides a far more accurate picture of medical board efforts to "protect the public". The only state agencies delegated with the authority to regulate the practice of medicine in each and every state have always been missing-in-action when questionable patient care events occur. That is why hospitals are the only place in America where an accidental death receives NO immediate review by a source of regulatory authority, and everyone continues to passively accept that sad fact.

A North Carolina physician was appointed to that state's medical board in 2003, the year after that litigation Center event. That physician became Medical Board President in 2007–2008, and earlier had become involved with the Federation of State Medical Boards in 2005. That earlier committee involvement led to that North Carolina physician being elected to the FSMB Board of Directors in 2008 and ultimately to become the Federation's Chairperson for 2011-12.

Federation of State Medical Boards (FSMB)

The Federation of State Medical Boards was established in 1912 is a national nonprofit organization representing 70 medical and osteopathic boards within the United States and its territories. Over the course of a century the FSMB has grown from a small annual gathering of state board executive officers with no permanent staff or headquarters to a vibrant national organization staffed by nearly 200 employees in the Dallas Texas area.

The Federation of State Medical Boards is a leader in medical regulation, serving as an innovative catalyst for effective policy and standards. FSMB leads by promoting excellence in medical practice, licensure, and regulation as a national resource and voice on behalf of state medical boards in their protection of the public. FSMB, an organization of state medical boards, embraces these equally important values: public protection, leadership, integrity, excellence, and commitment to service. Will someone ever dare FSMB to provide hard evidence of the above?

International Association of Medical Regulatory Authorities

The Federation of State Medical Boards of the United States, under contract with the US Department of Health and Human Services, planned and conducted the first international conference on medical regulation at a meeting in Washington DC in May 1994. Representatives of Australia, Canada, Ireland, New Zealand, South Africa, the United Kingdom, and the United States were in attendance along with observers from Egypt, Israel, Mexico and Taiwan.

IAMRA membership list includes over thirty-five national agencies and some of those nations listed include Ghana, India, Indonesia, Kenya, Korea, Malaysia, Nigeria, Pakistan, Sudan, and The Gambia.

The 10th biennial international conference on medical regulation was held in Philadelphia, Pennsylvania in September 2012.

Response: So the Federation of State Medical Boards and the Department of Health and Human Services felt, almost twenty years ago, and about the time that Harvard School of Public Health researchers were estimating that some 98,000 needless hospital deaths were occurring annually in our hospitals, that all of our state medical examining boards were doing such a wonderful job in protecting the public, the world could benefit from having an International Association of Medical Regulatory Authorities (note the words *Association* and *regulatory authorities* in that title).

People who complain about the obvious deficiencies in our Health Care Delivery System, and most people do complain, need to recognize the need to connect the dots regarding all of those who say they are working to make things better in health care, and what the evidence clearly demonstrates. Also, a reminder that I am not making any of this up, but just using their own words to illustrate the reality of our dysfunctional Health Care Delivery System.

Additional Insight

This brief, but insightful, article appeared in the Greenville News in the early 90s, and about the time the FSMB was helping to create the IAMRA.

Doctors told us not to tamper with lawsuit witnesses.

South Carolina doctors and their primary insurer will be charged with obstructing justice if they're caught tampering with witnesses in medical malpractice lawsuits from now on. Those who contact witnesses in court cases will risk criminal charges, the US Justice Department warned this week after privately notifying the President-elect of the South Carolina Medical Association that he won't be indicted for talking to a witness last fall.

But that President-elect of the State Medical Association came dangerously close to criminal charges when he urged another doctor to downplay a patient's injuries in court, a letter from federal prosecutors suggests. A similar letter was mailed to the legal counsel for the manager of the Joint Underwriting Association, which insures most doctors in this state. That manager also is the executive director of the patient's compensation fund, which helps pay malpractice verdicts that exceed the Association's $100,000 coverage limit.

The U.S. Attorney confirmed that both men are no longer criminal targets but have been put on notice that federal authorities consider any attempt to improperly influence testimony a very serious violation of law and will be alert to any attempts to cross the lines we have laid down.

The US Justice Department provided that medical society President-elect and that manager of the Joint Underwriting Association, through their attorneys, some stern guidance about the legality of approaching witnesses.

Both men were called before the grand jury after a federal judge heard that they might have tried to influence a doctor's testimony in a $3 million lawsuit. The U.S. Attorney refused to disclose the current contents of letters, but he said we made it clear what is legal and what is not in terms of connecting witnesses in any court case.

In the particular instance investigated by the grand jury, based on those facts and circumstances, there was not an illegal attempt to influence a witness under the strict interpretation of the law. We have to consider these things on a case-by-case basis.

Justice Department officials said they expected the medical society President-elect and the manager of the Joint Underwriting Association to spread the word throughout their organizations, however, since both testified in sworn depositions that contacting witnesses has been a common practice for the two associations because of their mutual interest in holding cost of malpractice litigation down.

According to the manager of the Joint Underwriting Association's sworn statement, at least 1000 South Carolina physicians had volunteered to talk to witnesses in such cases, but their purpose is to educate, not intimidate.

Everything contained thus far in this chapter was obtained from sources open to the public. At the same time, nothing contained thus far in this chapter would ever see the light of day within any component of the Quality of Health Care Army of Experts.

I have over 50 years' experience in our nation's Health Care Delivery System, and I know that the factual material contained in this chapter thus far raises questions, important question, that are not only never asked, but they are also never considered to be asked. Furthermore, the few people who might be capable of asking those important questions would never be allowed to ask them, and even if allowed to ask, they would lack the *authority* sufficient to receive meaningful answers.

Bill's parents merely represent the tip of the tip of the medical malpractice iceberg. And the needless hospital death fiasco completely ignores the much-larger dilemma of those patients who are or have received questionable patient care and lived to tell the tale. How did our Health Care Delivery System come to be such a chaotic mess?

A Brief History of Health Care

Our Health Care Delivery System began the first day a *man* stepped ashore and said, "I am a doctor, and I treat patients." Dr. Benjamin Rush signed the Declaration of Independence in 1776 and he was only one of the estimated 3,500 "doctors" in those days. But only 1 in 10 of those "doctors" had obtained a medical degree from a recognized school of medicine.

Doctors initially ruled themselves until Organized Medicine began to become "organized", and because all doctors are human, and all humans make mistakes, the problem of questionable patient care is, and always will be, an integral part of the "practice of medicine". Therefore, since doctors (all doctors) will make mistakes, what means are there to respond to those inevitable medical mistakes?

Three Potential Systems
NEW JERSEY LAW REVISION COMMISSION
FINAL REPORT Relating to
MEDICAL PEER REVIEW PRIVILEGE

Medical peer review is a process whereby doctors evaluate the quality of work done by their colleagues, to determine compliance with accepted health care standards. This self-regulatory procedure provides quality assurance for the medical community by fostering standardization of appropriate medical procedures and by policing caregivers who could pose risks to patients. The rationale for the process is efficiency: working doctors are best situated to judge the competence of other working doctors because they regularly see each other's work and possess the relevant expertise to evaluate it.

A peer review committee typically performs two functions: the initial process of credentialing (reviewing a doctor's qualifications and recommending whether the doctor should be granted privileges at the hospital), and ongoing review of a doctor's work within the hospital. Peer review is one of the chief means of monitoring the quality of doctors' work; the other two are state licensing board disciplinary action and tort law medical malpractice. Ideally, effective peer review should decrease the number of medical malpractice events and improve overall health care. Doctors, courts, and critics recognize the review process as an efficient means of professional self-regulation. "[P]eer review has become widely accepted as the primary means to weed out low quality physicians and to identify and offer assistance to physicians whose skills need to be enhanced in certain areas." Susan O. Scheutzow, "State Medical Peer Review: High Cost but No Benefit—Is it Time for a Change?", 25 *Am. J. L. & Med.* 7, 15 (1999).

Fundamentals of the review of questionable patient care

These two paragraphs are loaded with what anyone who thinks they, or a loved one has been harmed by medical care needs to know. There are now, and long have been three, only three, *potential systems* for the review of questionable patient care. Sadly, each one of those potential systems, each for its own reason, has been miserable failures.

"Ideally, effective peer review should decrease the number of medical malpractice events and improve overall health care." Ideally, our nation should also not be forced to deal with an estimated 200,000 needless hospital deaths annually for the last 20 years. Ideal medical peer review, except for a few isolated incidents, has been a figment of Organized Medicine's imagination, and a tool of their enormous PR. Medical peer review has all of the substance of fog. I know that to be true, and I can prove it.

I served on a hospital Formal Medical Peer Review Committee in 1976 that took all of the hospital privileges away from a general surgeon who had been in practice in Madison, Wisconsin for about 25 years. This surgeon had been grandfathered into having surgical privileges involving thoracic surgery, vascular surgery, and obstetrical surgery. Unfortunately, that surgeon was having a significantly higher rate of morbidity and mortality complications because he was continuing to use outdated surgical techniques.

I believe one of the major reasons why this surgeon was brought before a medical staff peer review committee was because he had practiced so long in the city in his solo practice and had never established a support group within his fellow practitioner circle.

Medical peer review, the few times it might take place, rarely involves a doctor well positioned with the in-crowd. Isolated, or fringe members of their local medical community are far more susceptible to being reviewed, should the need arise.

Our Peer Review Committee had no guidelines and no framework to function by, but I believe a majority of that committee's members made the correct decision in removing all of that surgeon's hospital privileges because he gave every indication that he saw no need in his making any changes in how he treated his patients or why several of his patient care techniques should be considered outdated.

That surgeon immediately sued the hospital and each individual member of that Review Committee for $1 million each back when $1 million was big money. My wife's response was, "What have you got yourself involved in now?" Fortunately, very shortly thereafter a judge denied his suit on the grounds that a hospital medical staff had the right to utilize the peer-reviewed process. That ruling meant I could keep my house.

The question that should be asked, and never is, is does meaningful medical peer review take place within hospital medical staff proceedings on a regular basis throughout our health care system? After all, the New Jersey Law Revision Commission said, "Medical peer review is a process whereby doctors evaluate the quality of work done by their colleagues, in order to determine compliance with accepted health care standards." But unfortunately, the answer to, does meaningful medical peer review take place, is, No! Simply put, hospital medical staff peer view occurs about as often as snowfalls in New Orleans?

I can provide any state governor and state legislature with a very simple test that could determine the degree of meaningful medical peer review in every hospital in any state and that process could be rapidly executed. Of course, such a test could only be performed if sufficient authority could be provided. Fortunately, this test would not require piercing of the medical peer review veil of secrecy. This last remark, however, brings up another important point regarding medical peer review.

Health Care Quality Improvement Act of 1986 was passed by Congress with the intent to protect peer review bodies from private money damage liability, and because Organized Medicine said that doctors could not feel free to speak about the patient care of other doctors unless such reports were made in complete secrecy.

I however believe Organized Medicine had an additional reason to seek Congressional passage of an act that would make medical peer review secret, and they were successful in obtaining their ultimate goal. All fifty state legislatures, like lemmings, rapidly followed Congress and now medical peer review is both secret and sacrosanct throughout our nation's hospitals. Unfortunately, due to that impregnable veil of secrecy, meaningful medical peer review's mere existence is left to one's reliance on our Medical Profession's veracity. Nonetheless, every hospital medical staff leader would respond, if queried, "Certainly we have medical peer review. But I would have to kill you if I told you about it because medical peer review is secret."

I repeat; I can provide any governor and any state legislature with a simple test that would demonstrate rapidly that medical peer review is for all practical purposes nonexistent in any of their state's hospitals. I welcome the challenge to provide such a test, but I am not optimistic that I will ever be able to find a governor or state legislature who might want to know the truth about medical peer review in their state's hospitals. Their citizens would probably like to know, but that is an entirely different matter.

Now, go back and slowly reread those first two paragraphs taken from the New Jersey Law Revision Commission Report and see if you have EVER seen the slightest indication that meaningful medical peer review takes place in the hospital medical staff at the hospital or hospitals near you. I know how and where to look, and I can tell you, medical peer review has all of the substance of fog.

State legislatures deserve much of the blame for the ability of hospital medical staff to conduct their professional-regulatory affairs behind closed doors. Congress, unwittingly by the ill-conceived HCQIA-86, gave each state the cover to allow them to make peer review secret. That, plus the periodic efforts to be led by the state components of Organized Medicine to enact Tort Reform measures that consistently increase the doctor's leverage in medical litigation cases go to make it almost impossible for a patient harmed by medical care to have a fair chance in the Sue or Forget It world of medical malpractice litigation.

Medical Malpractice Tort Reform

In early March 2004 I was eagerly awaiting the arrival of the first copies of my first published book, First, Do No Harm like an expectant father when I noticed in the local paper that a South Carolina Senate Judiciary Subcommittee would be holding a closed hearing regarding tort reform. I attended that closed hearing and joined a gallery of approximately 20 individuals. Their meeting began with about five or six Senators seated around the table, and 2-3 additional Senators joined them while the meeting was in progress. Watching those Senators seeking to reconcile their widely divergent viewpoints regarding tort reform was like watching middle-aged men herd cats.

At the conclusion of that meeting, and after all of the Senators had left, and I was alone in the gallery I approach the Senate Judiciary Committee's Legal Counsel and asked him, "How do you maintain your sanity?" However, there was something beneficial that came out of that chaotic meeting for their future considerations.

Tort reform has two distinctly different aspects, commercial and industrial tort reform, and medical malpractice tort reform. Just as our health care system has two distinctly different aspects, Cost & Access and Health Care Delivery System, all considerations of tort reform, to be effective, must recognize and proceed with that most important understanding. Following that meeting both Houses of the South Carolina Legislature attempting to deal with tort reform issues had their respective subcommittees separate the two distinctly different aspects of tort reform, and later combine those efforts into a final, legislative bill.

Medical malpractice tort reform, in my opinion, has been receiving far more consideration during the last decade than it deserves. Medical malpractice tort reform is the caboose of the medical malpractice litigation system, and that tort reform aspect can only become viable IF the plaintiff (patient) wins their case against the doctor, which only occurs statistically in about one out of ten medical malpractice trials. Medical malpractice tort reform is no magic wand, and it never has been.

This book, so far, reads as though I have a vendetta toward the medical profession, and that is not true. My concern is that the medical profession, and my profession, dentistry, have failed in their responsibilities to conduct themselves as true professions. One of the absolutes necessary to be a true professional is self-regulation of its members (medical peer review), and sadly, in that responsibility both professions are miserable failures. That fact is the root cause of all of the shortcomings of the healing arts profession. Thus, hopefully, the expertise of another expert's opinion will support the understanding that I am not out to kill the medical profession.

Joint Commission

Joint Commission was created in 1950 by the combined efforts of the AMA, American College of Surgeons, Americana College of Physicians, and the American Hospital Association. But the Joint Commission achieved their power, and commanding influence in 1965 with the creation of Medicare and Medicaid, and the need for some entity to "certify hospitals" for eligibility to receive Medicare reimbursement, and Congress, and almost every state, chose the Joint Commission to fulfill that necessary chore.

I have long considered the Joint Commission to be one of the greatest frauds perpetrated on the public, and not just because of their survey team's disrespectful, and unprofessional response to Agnes, therefore I offer a few examples of the true nature of the Joint Commission.

Joint Commission 1988 Wall Street Journal

Walt Bogdanich, writing in a front-page article, gave a description of the Joint Commission that was a far cry from Organized Medicine's description of their benevolent standard-bearer and dispenser of the hospital world's highest "seal of approval." He claimed that the Joint Commission's standard operating procedure at that time was to accept virtually every hospital that applied for accreditation. In addition, the Joint Commission rarely, if ever, disciplined or punished hospitals that violated its standards. Perhaps, suggested Bogdanich, that was because the commission's multi-million-dollar budget was primarily covered by hospital fees for accreditation.

At that time, hospitals were given at least a one-month advance notice of an on-site inspection, and the results of that inspection were kept confidential. Furthermore, for a hefty sum, the commission sold consultant packages advising hospitals how to pass an inspection.

A survey of the Joint Commission data for the period 1986 to 1988 showed that of 5,208 accredited hospitals, 51% did not have adequate procedures for reviewing surgery; 56% did not properly monitor or evaluate how well the medical staff in different departments gave care; and more than 40% were cited for violations of safety standards while keeping their accreditation. As Bogdanich pointed out, one New York hospital was closed by the state for violations immediately after it had been accredited by the Joint Commission. Shortly thereafter, New York State decided to stop using the Joint Commission to accredit its hospitals.

Following the adverse publicity, the Joint Commission promised to reform. New committees were formed. New people took office. New standards for patient safety and medical/healthcare error reduction in hospitals were written. It was promised that a random, unannounced inspection policy would be implemented. Twenty

  member standards review task force was formed to pinpoint where accreditation standards were most relevant to the safety and quality of patient care and to recommend the elimination or modification of standards that did not contribute to good patient care. Press releases trumpeted new standards for office-based surgeries, for patient restraint, for treatment of specific diseases, and a dozen other projects.

Joint Commission, "We have to demonstrate that we're fair, equitable, and sensitive and that we're not policemen."

2002 Chicago Tribune

Reporters Michael Berens and Bruce Japsen did another in-depth investigation of the organization. They found even more shocking flaws in the system, which now involves fewer hospitals 4,800, but more care facilities 14,000. The cost of being accredited has risen to $40,000 and the pre-investigation consultation cost $10,000. Instead of giving hospitals a month of lead time before inspections, the commission now gives them three months. Joint Commission allows hospitals to choose the patient files to be reviewed; obviously, these will all be success stories with happy endings.

The fact is that the Joint Commission is accountable to no one—not to government or to patients—and this lack of accountability has allowed it to grow out of control. After more than 50 years of being the profession's answer to self-regulation and 40 years of being the federal government's seal of approval for Medicare, the Joint Commission has developed cracks in its wall of secrecy that are finally allowing the public a glance at what regulation and standardization of the profession by the profession amounts to.

For instance, the Joint Commission has created a list of "sentinel events" that are supposed to act like smoke detectors. Any one event will bring the Joint Commission investigators to a hospital. They define a sentinel event is "an unexpected occurrence involving death or serious physical or psychological injury."

A recent sentinel event occurred at Children's Hospital in St. Louis when 90 cases of salmonella poisoning were reported. The kitchen was shut down for 10 days while an investigation was conducted. Once the kitchen was cleaned and a couple of food handlers were dismissed, the investigation ended. Will the incident show up in the Joint Commission's records? Incredibly, since 1995, the Joint Commission has documented only 12 cases of preventable hospital-borne infections from the thousands of healthcare facilities it monitors.

In 2002, infections in a Florida hospital caused eighteen deaths and brought out more than 100 litigants against the medical center. All of the litigants had undergone cardiac surgery and had become disabled as a result of infection. The Joint Commission's sent investigators, but their findings were withheld from those who were infected. "If we want any modicum of cooperation from the hospitals, they have to feel we're not going to put investigative findings right out on the street," said the Joint Commission president, Dr. Dennis O' Leary. One of the litigants responded, "It's outrageous. This infection has destroyed my life, but I'm being treated like I'm the bad guy."

My response:

Twenty years after Agnes' story, and nothing has changed. Organized Medicine, at every level, national, state, and local demonstrate that between the Code of Silence, and Dr. Palmisano's definition of medical malpractice as being patient care beneath the standard of care SET BY THE LAW, and there is NO medical malpractice without expert witness testimony, and doctors can't risk becoming an expert witness because of the code of silence, the failure of all professionalism is assured.

My latest success:

2014 Ali, a young Muslim in Southern California had a need for a surgical expert witness. Ali had just graduated from law school, or was near graduation when he first contacted me, and asked if I would review the records of his recent, highly questionable oral surgery, and I said I would. I had briefly mentioned my service as a plaintiff's expert witness for Ali in the Foreword.

Ali had a slight, lower jaw deformity that required a simple, mandibular set-back, and slight readjustment of his dental mid-line, and his surgeon had consent from Ali, prior to his surgery for just such a relatively simple, horizontal reposition of his lower jaw. There were two problems with this straight-forward treatment plan.

Ali had chosen this particular oral surgeon because he advertised and reported himself to be a dual-degree (MD/DDDS) surgeon, and therefore Ali considered him to be of a superiorly qualified surgeon. That was not the case. His surgeon had obtained his "medical degree" from a Caribbean diploma-mill, as I was to find out, so had about 3 dozen other "oral surgeons" throughout the country.

Secondly, Ali's surgeon, for reasons unknown in Ali's surgical records, had changed the original treatment plan to now include a vertical dimension change, plus the necessary horizontal change, and that additional surgery created great, and unnecessary post-surgical problems, that resulted in great harm to Ali.

I told Ali, and his highly qualified trial attorney, that I did consider that his records clearly indicated he had been harmed by negligent care, and that I felt qualified to testify as an expert witness on his behalf if, and when necessary. Malpractice litigation moves very slowly, and three years after first being sought, Ali and his attorney contacted me with their great, and urgent need.

2017 Ali's surgeon's defense attorneys approached the trial judge with a claim that Ali and his attorney had shown no evidence of a viable claim of negligence on the part of their client, and therefore request that the trial judge dismiss the case entirely. Fortunately, Ali and his attorney were given an opportunity to demonstrate justification for their claim of negligence, and they called me.

I produced the **DECLARATION OF IRA WILLIAMS, D.D.S.** that consisted of seven legal-size pages, and over 2700 words that offered a detailed depiction of every sub-standard act committed by his surgeon, and every cause of negligent harm suffered by Ali.

Good News:

Ali, and his attorney called me to say that the judge had accepted my Declaration, and therefore the surgeon, and his attorneys, and his insurance company had settled the case in full. Also, I felt that I could consider myself as being the oldest, successful Plaintiff's (patient's) surgical expert witness in the country.

Bad News:

MICRA-75: That stands for MICKEY MOUSE—No, I'm sorry. It stands for: **Medical Injury Compensation Reform Act-1975** passed by the California Legislature that year that set the cap for malpractice payments at 250,000, and 42 years later it was still 250,000. Medical malpractice is adjudicated in state civil courts, and by state legislative regulations, and every state legislature has systematically favored the healing arts professions at their behest.

Furthermore, Congress passed the Health Care Quality Improvement Act-1986 (HCQIA-86), and with no true standing in state matters, made medical peer review *secret*, again at the behest of Organized Medicine, and within a very few years, all fifty state legislatures made medical peer review secret.

So, Ali won his case, and the California Legislature made it possible for the surgeon's insurance company to pay Ali in 1975 dollars. Ain't Government grand!

The System is Broken

Experts have agreed for decades; the HCDS is broken! I consider "broken" to be a poor word for such a critical understanding, but it certainly gets the point across – the healthcare system that is going to reach out and grab you, and every person you hold near and dear to your heart, is, and has always been "broken".

But saying the HCDS is broken is not sufficient. What has been missing in the litany of evidence of multiple failures within that "system" has been scant discussions regarding How, and Why that system is, and has always been broken.

First, I will share a historical timeline of best-known evidence of the HCDS being broken for the past 3 decades.

1985. Drs. Brennan and Leape, as co-leaders of a team of experts from the Harvard School of Public Health began a 4-year study of individual patient records in hospitals in Upstate New York, and only two years after Agnes' disgraceful medical malpractice panel that had judged her two doctors to have provided her with negligent care.

1989. The Brennan & Leape team would announce that during, by far the largest study of its kind, they now estimated 98,000 Needless Hospital Deaths annually, or 268/day. Their announcement in the New England Journal of Medicine had all of the impact of a tree falling in an empty forest.

1999. Institute of Medicine (IOM), now National Academy of Medicine (NAM) published the now famous or infamous report; To Err Is Human, and that report continues to receive great, and in my opinion, unfounded acclaim. My disdain for that report is based upon two critical inclusions in the first few pages.

That report was the work-product of two large committees, and early in the report it is noted that "some committee members thought the "fragmented nature of the health care delivery system *or non-system* to some observers—" Page 1

IF the current HCDS is, in fact, a non-system, everything the members of those two committees were doing should have stopped, and their efforts redirected.

SYSTEM, that word, has critical meaning; it implies the coordinated functioning of multiple components collaborating in a *systematic manner*. Later, in this timeline format, I will provide evidence that I have been trying for the past decade to convince the army of Quality of Care and Patient Safety experts that one of the two major reasons why, and how the current HCDS is broken is the fact that all of those experts, for the past 3 decades have ignored the fact that this thing everyone has been calling a "system" has always been devoid of any systematic characteristics.

To Err Is Human other, devaluing factor is the early promise made in that report that clearly demonstrates the complete fallacy of the entire report.

"Concluding that the know-how already exists to prevent many of these mistakes, the report sets as a minimum goal a 50 percent reduction in errors over the next five years." Page 2

Every <u>new</u> estimate of Needless Hospital Deaths offered in the coming years was greater than all previous estimates, or better said, every new estimate kept getting greater until.

2016 Medical Errors are the 3rd leading cause of deaths in the U.S. behind heart disease and cancer, as reported by Dr. Marty Makary, and a co-author. Still, not an eye blinked in DC or any state capital in response to that grim disclosure.

Also, little is said about To Err Is Human, the book, being the first in a series of 6 books: the second book, and the series sharing the same name, Crossing the Quality Chasm. I reviewed all 6 books and found that they offer 53 Recommendations presumably to contribute to the efforts to improve the quality of care and patient safety. They are, in my opinion, bureaucratic nonsense, and offer no evidence of moving the needle in a positive direction toward their goal. The proof: I repeat, every new estimate of Needless Hospital Deaths has been greater than all previous estimates for the past 3 decades. But there is more.

My Bookends refer to personal efforts in 2010-11, and 2019-20 primarily because of the persons of highest authority I sought to engage with, and share my concerns, and expertise.

2010 Three Events:

"Even if we had a cure for cancer, we couldn't get it to the people because the current system is broken!" Dr. Spence Taylor, Chairman of the Committee seeking to establish a new medical school in Greenville SC. Greenville Journal, April.

MISDIAGNOSED! WHY CURRENT HEALTH CARE CHANGE IS MALPRACTICE, my 2nd book was published in September.

Nikki Haley was successfully elected Governor and said she would listen to anyone seeking to speak with her in November.

2011: Two Events

"There's no question that our nation's healthcare system is broken." Ingo Angermeier, President/CEO, Spartanburg Regional Hospital, and former President, South Carolina Hospital Association. Greenville Magazine, April.

Governor Nikki Haley provided me with a 10-minute face-to-face meeting in August. I first showed her my back-to-back copies of Dr. Taylor's and Ingo's quotes, and a copy of my latest book, *MISDIAGNOSED!* I then told her that I could provide her with a detailed picture of her State's HCDS. She made no comment, and no offer to meet again.

2013. Governor Haley sent word she could not accept my offer, but no reason given, even though she had published a book the year she was elected Governor entitled, *Can't Is Not An Option*. Apparently, "can't" was her only option regarding the SC HCDS.

2020: Three Events

CMS Director Verma provided me with contact to her office at a face-to-face meeting in December 2019.

2021. I Met with CMS Chief of Medical Staff Dr. Shari Ling, and other staff members at CMS Baltimore Headquarters for 1 hour on March 5th, and I established Contact with CMS Innovation Center Director Brad Smith in May.

My email message to Director Verma, Dr. Ling, and Director Smith in June contained the following: I can provide a process for how to begin to create a 21st century Healthcare Delivery System (doctors, hospitals, and surgery centers). NO response has been received.

So, during a ten year span my offer to contribute to the efforts to make your and your loved one's HCDS far better have been rejected, first by then SC Governor Nikki Haley, and more recently by CMS Director Verma, and CMS Innovation Center Director Smith, all with NO reason given. But back to why the current HCDS is and has always been broken.

The Two Greatest HCDS Mistakes

System is devoid of any systematic characteristics. It is almost impossible to write or speak about HEALTHCARE without being compelled to use the word *system*. Yet every time that word is used regarding HEALTHCARE, the user is misleading themselves, and any potential audience. Still, none, and I do mean none, of the Quality of Care and Patient Safety army of experts, including the five Federally created Quality of

Care agencies created by Congress, beginning in 1970, have ever focused on that critically important issue.

Other Great HCDS Mistake

1. All medical care is local. You get sick or injured, and you will receive local medical care.

2. States license doctors, hospitals, and surgery centers.

I am left with only one logical conclusion; Each state is responsible to create and maintain an effective HCDS for its citizens, and no governor or state legislator, past or present, has ever recognized, and sought to act on that responsibility. And none of the Federal Quality of Care Agencies have ever recognized or considered each state's responsibility for their HCDS.

2016 I became aware that two of those Federal Quality of Care Agencies had scheduled all-day meetings during the same week in, or near D.C., and I made plans to attend both meetings, and hand-deliver an offer-letter to each President/Director.

Dr. Ira E. Williams
My address
September 26, 2016

September 28, 2016

<u>Victor J. Dzau, President</u>
National Academy of Medicine

<u>Andrew Bindman, MD, Director</u>
Agency for Healthcare Research and Quality

*Subject: **The Two Greatest Healthcare Mistakes***

Medical errors are now considered to be the 3rd leading cause of deaths in the U.S., and every new estimate of needless hospital deaths has been greater than all previous estimates for the past quarter century, and since Brennan & Leape (1990).

There are reasons why no discernable progress has been made in improving the quality of healthcare and patient safety, and I suggest that many of those reasons can be found in;

The Two Greatest Healthcare Mistakes that have been unrecognized or ignored.

I am requesting The National Academy of Medicine permit me to present.

- The Two Greatest Healthcare Mistakes
- A 3-step process on how to begin to create a 21st century healthcare delivery system.

In those presentations I will identify and describe in detail what has always been missing in the efforts to improve the quality of healthcare and patient safety.

Semmelweis did not create the fact that IF doctors washed their hands, and sterilized their instruments fewer patients would needlessly die. He recognized, tested, and proved the life-saving value of those patient-care facts, but his patient-care advancements were not accepted by the medical leadership of his day.

I did not create the facts that support the understanding of the Two Greatest Healthcare Mistakes, and how recognition of those mistakes can provide the means to begin to create a 21st century healthcare delivery system. I can only hope that my request will not receive a similar response as that received by Semmelweis, first in Vienna, and later in Budapest.

Experts should not only be challenged, but they should seek to be challenged.

Sincerely,
Ira E. Williams, D.D.S.

Since both letters were identical, I combined the headings. Like SC Governor Haley, both Agency heads were unimpressed, and never responded in any manner. Sadly, I have found the Quality of Care and Patient Safety experts to collectively, and individually have "bear-trap minds, and all of them are closed." Each expert not only should be challenged, because no expert knows everything that needs to be considered, and therefore, every expert should seek to be challenged.

It has long been my belief that it will continue to impossible to begin to create a far better HCDS for our Nation, until, and unless those Two Greatest Mistakes are recognized, and included in every effort.

Why the current HCDS is broken, in my opinion, is the failure to recognize those two great mistakes.

How is the HCDS Broken

Agnes' story, and particularly the unprofessional hospital medical staff peer review, followed by the disgraceful Joint Commission, and Wisconsin medical malpractice panel system tells you everything you need to know about How the HCDS is broken.

The vast majority of all patient care is accepted, and that is all it needs to be. Most doctors are average, at best, and far too many patients are their own worst enemy regarding their care for their body, therefore when a person receives medical care with no discernable problems, the system is assumed to have "worked".

When individual patient care falls beneath an acceptable standard of care, and becomes questionable care, that is where the system has always failed. The medical profession has always failed its professional responsibility to attempt to self-regulate its members, and has, instead, left the public with Sue or Forget It, followed by attempting to destroy every patient's expert witness with the Code of Silence.

2007. I created The Two Missing Links of Medical Malpractice, and also had it produced in audio CD form. I was able to visualize this concept of relating the practice of medicine to the process of learning to fly a single-engine airplane due to my 13-

year experience as a USAF navigator, and my obtaining, and using a private pilot's license. I believe this thought paper offers an insightful way to hopefully better understand the related aspects of doctors attempting to treat the medical needs of their patients.

The Two Missing Links of Medical Malpractice
Dr. Ira Williams

A crisis is defined as a period of instability. The medical malpractice crisis, now in its fourth decade of social instability, displays no real evidence of reaching a solution. Dr. Ira Williams, author of *First, Do No Harm, The Cure for Medical Malpractice* offers a compelling clarification of the fundamental cause of that ongoing dilemma, **The Two Missing Links of Medical Malpractice.**

"Medical malpractice, is it, or isn't it? How can we know?" Let me open with a poorly recognized fact, which hopefully will crystallize the immense depth of this problem. I will use three unfortunate events which could occur in any community in our nation tomorrow; however, these are three unfortunate events which did occur at different times in my community.

First Event: A construction worker is accidentally killed at the worksite. OSHA investigators are on the scene within hours.

Second Event: A single engine airplane crashes on takeoff. Both occupants walked away with only slight injuries. FAA investigators are at the site within hours.

Third Event: A 27-year-old slender, healthy wife and mother enters the hospital OR for minor knee surgery under local anesthesia. She's injected once in the upper thigh on the front and once in the buttocks. Within minutes she suffered a catastrophic system collapse, and within a few additional minutes she was clinically dead. No investigators from any regulatory body ever appeared at the site of that tragedy. The widowed husband was forced to sue the doctors in order to find out what happened. On the third anniversary of her death a lay jury returned a verdict of no negligence. The doctors had won another court case. Two very significant factors must be gained from that tragic story.

First, hospitals are probably the only site in America where an accidental death can occur and receive no regulatory in-depth investigation. How frightening!

Second, the practice of medicine is probably the least regulated economic activity in America today.

Doctors are the best judge of other doctors, but doctors do not know how to judge other doctors. Medical malpractice happens. Doctors are only human, and all humans make mistakes. Even the best doctors make mistakes. The big problem is not that medical malpractice happens, it's inevitable. The big problem is our medical profession's failure to fairly judge questionable patient care within their profession. The issue should not be medical malpractice. The issue is questionable patient care and more specifically how can doctors fairly judge questionable patient care?

History plays an important part in understanding medical malpractice. Medical malpractice is a cultural event and cultural events do not take place in a vacuum. Throughout American history the practice of medicine has been a state regulated activity, and one might add, a very poorly regulated activity. For over 150 years almost all in-depth reviews of questionable patient care have occurred before a judge, and lay, or non-medical jury.

Medical malpractice first became a recognized crisis in the mid-1800s and that crisis, like the morning and evening tide, has fluctuated within our society ever since. The obvious root cause of that malpractice crisis has remained puzzlingly obscure to everyone.

Doctors are by far the best judge of other doctors and therefore they should be the best judge of questionable patient care. That makes sense. But doctors have never created a system whereby they can fairly judge other doctors regarding questionable patient care.

Sometimes the obvious escapes notice. Doctors, our medical profession, has not one but two gigantic failures lurking in our otherwise marvelous history of modern medicine.

Failure number 1: *We have never created a system whereby doctors can fairly judge the questionable patient care of another doctor without attorneys, courts, and juries.*

Failure number 2: *We can provide zero evidence that our learned profession has even made a determined effort to create such a system.*

To understand the cause of those two failures you must understand the basic elements of all medical care. From a tonsillectomy to a heart transplant, all medical treatments have several common, basic elements. Three of those basic elements are:

1. Science
2. Art
3. Standard of Care

Doctors, all doctors, are taught the *science of medicine*. Medical schools teach the science of medicine and turn non-doctors into doctors. Doctors, all doctors, provide the *art of medicine*. More precisely, each doctor provides his or her personal art of medicine to each patient they treat. Therefore, each patient is a fresh canvas demonstrating that doctor's art of medicine.

The perfect analogy for the practice of medicine is a pilot flying a single engine airplane. Each student pilot is taught the science of flying an airplane. Each pilot, student, or graduate pilot provides their personal art of flying an airplane each time they take off and hopefully land safely. The exact same combination of science and art occurs each and every time a doctor treats a patient.

This basic understanding exposes a major component of the medical malpractice dilemma and that is; all medical treatment is a combination of science and art. But the medical profession, as of today, has never been able to identify, define and more importantly judge the art of medicine. That fact, the medical profession's inability to identify, define and judge one of the two basic characteristics of every form of medical care is the **First Missing Link** in the medical malpractice crisis.

The Standard of Care is the Second Missing Link in the malpractice crisis.

Just as every form of medical care is a combination of science and art, every form of medical care has a standard of care automatically attached to it. A doctor cannot treat a patient in any manner without there being a standard of care associated with that treatment. The question is asked; "Doctor, you treated this patient, what was your standard of care for that treatment?"

What was the standard of care is the critical question, which must be answered in every review of questionable patient care. Now that I have identified the two-missing links in the medical malpractice crisis; One, finding the art of medicine and two, what is the standard of care, let's briefly review the current history of medical malpractice, or the better term, questionable patient care. As stated earlier, medical malpractice happens, but not all questionable patient care is medical malpractice. So, how can we judge what questionable patient care is medical malpractice and what questionable patient care is not?

Currently there are three different systems that potentially may be used for the review of questionable patient care.

First there are the state medical examining boards. Data from the Federation of State Medical Examining Boards show this system to rarely be used for the review of questionable patient care. The potential for such use does exist, but in name only.

Second there is medical peer review. Doctors review the patient care of other doctors. Peer review can occur at several levels of organized medicine, but the most effective system of medical peer review should occur at the hospital medical staff level.

Does medical peer review occur by hospital medical staffs? Probably not, because Congress and the state legislatures made medical peer review totally secret. Medical peer review is more secret than almost anything else nonmilitary. Yes, medical peer review does exist, but like fog, there is no discernible substance to medical peer review, and no identifiable benefit to society. Medical peer review and the state medical examining board's review of questionable patient care both essentially exist in name only.

Third is the obvious, medical malpractice litigation. The center of all public debate regarding questionable patient care. Sadly, if medical peer review functions properly it should result in far less malpractice litigation. So there exists three decidedly different systems with a potential ability to judge questionable patient care.

Number one, state medical examining boards are rarely if ever used to judge questionable patient care. Number two, medical peer review is ultra-secret and there is no evidence in any city or town that this system functions to society's benefit. And number three, malpractice litigation.

There are countless articles and books detailing the laundry list of failures associated with this system. Yet all three systems demand that the state board reviewers, medical peer review committee, and/or the civil court judge or jury create the medical standard of care they are to judge by.

And now for the central point of this discussion; the *AMA definition of medical malpractice is treatment beneath a standard of care set by the law*, their words not mine.

So where does that leave society? There can be no medical treatment given by a doctor to a patient without that treatment having a medical standard of care. Yet the AMA defines medical malpractice as treatment beneath a standard of care set by the law.

And people wonder why medical malpractice a major problem within our society for over 150 years has been. Doctors do not know how to judge other doctors. The root cause of the problem stops there.

Until and unless doctors create a system where-by they can fairly judge other doctors regarding questionable patient care, the medical malpractice crisis will continue to exist and continue to grow. Such a system whereby doctors can fairly judge other doctors without attorneys, courts and juries is far more attainable than imagined. Let's go back to the basics of all medical treatment.

Doctors are taught the science of medicine. Doctors provide the art of medicine. Just as water requires two hydrogen and one oxygen molecule, all medical treatment requires the science and the art of medicine to result in a standard of care.

A doctor's standard of care for every form of treatment he or she provides can only be found by reviewing those three elements in detail.

So how might one review the three basic elements of all medical care? The science of every form of medical treatment can be written identical to the format of a single engine airplane checklist.

No person should willingly submit to surgery performed by a doctor who was unable or unwilling to document the scientific elements of their personal standard of care for the planned surgical procedure.

Yet this is exactly what occurs and what our medical profession permits on a daily basis.

Doctors are never required to document the scientific elements of the standard of care they have been taught and use in the daily performance of their profession.

Yet the scientific elements of every medical standard of care are the center pole of any system of review of questionable patient care. You can't have one, medical treatment without the other, a standard of care.

Doctors created the medical malpractice litigation crisis by their failure to create a system whereby doctors, the best judges, could judge other doctors without attorneys, courts, and juries. Thus, society was left with "*sue or forget it*", and attorneys filled the vacuum the doctors created by their own failure.

The AMA states, "The primary cause of America's medical liability crisis is overzealous personal injury attorneys who put their pocketbooks before patients." Now ask yourself, if a person has surgery, and in time reasonable questions arise, that happens right, how, when, and where did an attorney create the problem? The AMA has no answer for that question.

Doctors are the best judge of other doctors, but doctors don't know how to judge other doctors. But since Congress, state legislatures, and the AMA think that medical malpractice is treatment beneath a standard of care set by the law then who cares?

Decades ago, doctors failed to recognize the fatal flaw they were creating by not creating a system of medical peer review which could complement the marvelous scientific achievements of their profession.

When doctors left society with *"sue or forget it"* they drove a stake into the heart of their own profession. Only a system of medical peer review fair to both doctor and patient can ever right that wrong.

Our medical profession must redefine the definition of medical malpractice to treatment beneath a standard of care set by doctors, and not the law.

Fourteen years later, I believe this thought paper has stood the test of time and conveys what was sorely missing in Agnes' story.

I can go into any hospital or medical center, and IF provided with sufficient delegated authority to request, and receive necessary information, I can demonstrate two different forms of unethical, and unprofessional behavior by members of the medical staff. Both types of unprofessional behavior are endemic to every hospital medical staff in America. One merely must know where and how to look.

But, enough about some of the multitude of failures of the current HCDS.

It's time to DREAM!

A 21st Century HCDS

How to begin:

First, each state's responsibility to create and maintain an effective HCDS must be recognized and accepted as fact. Bureaucratic Federal quality of care agencies have been promising real improvements in the quality of care and patient safety, and all they have been doing is demonstrating Einstein's definition of insanity.

Logic should demand that since all medical care is local, and state's license doctors, hospitals, and surgery centers, one's only conclusion must be each state is responsible for their HCDS.

Second, proving that the current HCDS is, and has always been, devoid of any systematic characteristics is far easier than may be anticipated, and that process should begin by asking and answering the question; where are we now, and how did we get here?

Identify every component that contributes to any state's current HCDS, and there are more of them than one might first imagine.

Next, identify <u>any</u> systematic collaboration between any of those components, and don't be surprised to find that they each function as though they each speak a different language. Thus, the absence of any true systematic characteristics will be finally revealed.

A process of identifying each component of the SC HCDS and seeking to identify any systematic characteristics within that "system" would have been the process used IF Governor Haley had accepted my 2011 offer and joined me in making Healthcare History.

A TEST: seek to find at least one person in any state capital who can claim the ability to describe, in detail, their state's current HCDS by identifying every component that contributes to that system and identifying any systematic collaboration. Good luck.

2017 Dr. Robert Pearl, former Chief of Staff of Kaiser Permanente for almost 2 decades, stated in his first book, *MISTREATED* that he likened the current HCDS to a 19th century cottage-industry. Most of the 19th century (1800-1899) doctors were still killing almost as many of their patients as they were able to benefit. Finally, late in that century Pasteur demonstrated via the Germ Theory that organisms too small to be seen by the naked eye were the source of those deaths, and his contribution helped open the door to what was slowly to become Modern Medicine. So, Dr. Pearl's dubious analogy is just one more example of current HCDS experts' failure to understand what should be obvious.

There is an urgent need to finally describe in great detail the current HCDS, and the fact that that obvious need has never been accomplished speaks volumes for why each new estimate of Needless Hospital Deaths have always been greater than all previous estimates. The numbers keep getting larger because the Quality of Care and Patient Safety army of experts are primarily led by doctors who continue to refuse to recognize that Needless Hospital Deaths are most likely due to medical (doctor) errors.

A summary

1989, ten years after Agnes' debacle, a team of Harvard School of Public Health led by two doctors, and after four years of research in Upstate New York hospitals, estimated there were 98,000 Needless Hospital Deaths (268/day) annually.

1999, ten more years later, Institute of Medicine (IOM) stated in their report To Err Is Human, "we have all we need to reduce that number (98,000) by 50% in 5 years." Tragically, IOM misspoke as every new estimate of Needless Hospital Deaths has been far greater than all previous estimates, and there is NO evidence that this deadly trend is being reversed.

2012 Dr. Makary's book UNACCOUNTABLE takes the reader behind the curtain, and into the Dark Side of hospital medical staffs, and his one-word title speaks volumes.

2016 Dr. Makary, and a co-author publish an article claiming that Medical Errors are the 3rd leading cause of deaths in the U.S., and no one seems to care.

And all of this was taking place while the AMA was determining that medical malpractice is harmful treatment beneath a standard of care *set by the law*. And those five federal Quality of Care and Patient Safety agencies continue demonstrating Einstein's definition of insanity, by doing the same thing over and over, while seeking a different solution.

Real Healthcare

What is Real Healthcare? A person in any of the 50 states, DC, or any of the territories becomes sick or injured sufficiently to require the service of a duly qualified and licensed doctor, and perhaps the need for such care to be provided in a hospital, or surgery center. In essence, the Healthcare Delivery System, or more precisely, where the Healthcare rubber meets the Healthcare Road. Naturally, in our long-established economic system, such care must be paid for, but only after the fact of that care. Unfortunately, for all concerned, the after-the-fact aspect of Healthcare has become the dominant aspect of the Healthcare System conundrum.

President Johnson, and a dominate Democratic Congress created the Medicare/Medicaid System in 1965-66, and instantly replaced doctors as the dominate force within those hospitals that chose to accept Medicare payments for their patient-care services in the future. Thus Cost & Access (payment after-the-fact) became, and has remained, the primary focus for all efforts to try to continually improve that System. So, what have been the results of Federal domination in Healthcare?

Eleven presidents, and 58 years of a Congress that is at least slightly changed every two years, and "they" still haven't gotten it right, and probably never will. How to pay for Healthcare after-the-fact ain't Healthcare! It is the economics of Healthcare, and therefore a critical part of the Healthcare conundrum, but to allow that aspect of Healthcare to become, and remain, the primary focus for the efforts to improve that System is letting the tail wag the dog, or as noted earlier, Selective Stupidity.

I have come to recognize what I term to be the 3 Greatest Healthcare Mistakes, but before I describe my vision of what has always been missing in the efforts to improve the Quality of Care and Patient Safety, I feel the need to provide some hopefully clarifying considerations.

Healthcare System is enormous, and complex, but I believe that anyone seeking a better understanding of that system needs to understand that such a task is not like coming to better understand brain surgery or nuclear physics. One should focus on the facts, and use Logic (2 + 2 = 4). Such a simplistic manner can be better understood by knowing that all of the Quality of Care and Patient Safety experts who have been promising to "make that system better" since the mid-1980s, and have so miserably failed in those efforts, have consistently failed to focus on the facts themselves. My challenge then is this, carefully consider my description of the 3 Greatest Healthcare Mistakes, while focusing on the facts, and then decide IF I have satisfied the Logic Test. One last point; these Mistakes should not be considered as 1-2-3, but rather as 1A-1B-1C, and joined at the hip, so to speak, as each supports the others.

Three Greatest Healthcare Mistakes

Mistake 1A

Allowing the Cost & Access aspect of Healthcare to become the primary focus on how to attempt to improve that System. Clinton-Care, Romney-Care, Obama-Care, and all the other never-ending pronouncements that, "this time we are really going to get it right!?" And, after over 50 years of such promises, they still haven't got it right. But more importantly, they have consistently treated the Healthcare Delivery System like an illegitimate child at a family reunion.

Our Nation's Healthcare System is comprised of two Equally Important Aspects, that are as different as "Boys" and "Girls", and those equally important aspects are Cost & Access, and Healthcare Delivery System, and there will never be any real progress in effectively making the current system far better without providing at least equal focus on the Delivery aspect of that System, and where Real Healthcare is provided. Presidents and Congresses have wasted billions of dollars, and decades of time, by thinking that they can improve the Quality of Care by throwing money at the problem. The Quality of Care can only be improved at the doctor/patient interface, where the Healthcare rubber meets the road. And I believe the weight of this Mistake can be better appreciated when included in the context of Mistakes 1B & 1C.

Mistake 1B

Each state is responsible for creating and maintaining an effective Healthcare Delivery System, and no governor, and no state legislator, past or present has ever recognized that responsibility. Focus on the Facts:

- **All medical care is local.**
- **States license hospitals, medical centers, and surgery centers.**
- **States license doctors (and nurses, bless the nurses).**
- **States license surgery centers and their professional staffs.**

Congress, beginning in 1970, and ending in 2010, has created 5 Federal Agencies tasked with providing means to improve the Quality of Care and Patient Safety within the current Healthcare System, and none of those Agencies have ever recognized, and incorporated into their efforts those Fundamental Facts regarding the delivery of care to every patient.

2011. I told newly elected SC Governor Nikki Haley, in a 10-min. face-to-face meeting that I could give her a detailed picture of her state's Healthcare Delivery System. She ended our very brief meeting abruptly, and never asked for more details. We could have made Healthcare history over a decade ago, but she couldn't go there, and no reason was ever given.

Two governors, two Lt. governors, two senators, the previous, and the current Congressman of my district, and countless state senators and house members have shown NO interest in confronting the well-established, and critically important failures in this, and every other state's Healthcare Delivery System, and again, no reason is ever given. All forms of the local media, Chamber of Commerce, and other civic organizations, and even the Greenville Library have chosen to ignore my efforts to create a dialogue regarding this matter, and I am left to wonder.

Your & Your Love One's Healthcare Delivery System is broken!
I know how to begin to create a far better system.
Does anyone care?

Mistake 1C

System. Just that one word, system. Those of us who speak or write about *healthcare* are rapidly compelled to add the word System, and each time we do, we are misleading ourselves, and any potential audience. The current System is, and has always been, a non-system, and the consistent refusal to recognized that Fact (there's that word again) is one of the fundamental flaws in all of the efforts to improve that System.

One should simply consider our body to better understand the word *system*. Our body functions using multiple systems; skeletal, muscular, vascular, nervous, etc. and indicating the *Systematic Collaboration of multiple elements.* Now contrast that understanding with any state's Healthcare Delivery System.

MISDIAGNOSED! Why Current Healthcare Change is Malpractice was my second book, self-published in 2010, and a copy of that book was given to Governor Haley at our very brief, and decidedly ineffective meeting. I described the SC Healthcare Delivery System in that book, by identifying each of the components that contribute in some way to the makeup of that System. I then began to recognize, because I have long, deep-seated experience in such a system, that each of those components function as if they each speak a different language, thus the non-system recognition.

The Test: Ask any governor if they, or any other person functioning within their state government can describe, in detail, their state's current Healthcare Delivery System by identifying each component that contributes to that system, and then identify any evidence of Systematic Collaboration between those components. Good luck!

Review and Reflect

Now review those 3 Healthcare Mistakes in concert, and recognize that both individually, and collectively, they have never been a part of all the efforts by that Quality of Care and Patient Safety army of experts during the 3 decades of efforts prior to COVID, or since. Does Selective Stupidity come to mind?

Therefore, I believe it will be impossible to ever begin to create a far better System unless the Fundamental Facts regarding each state's responsibility to create and maintain such a System are recognized and included. Real Healthcare takes place within each state's current System, and each state's current System is in critical need of fundamental change. And you should begin such change by asking and answering the 2-part question; where are we now, and how did we get here? You do that by describing in detail the current System and seeking to identify any evidence of Systematic Collaboration.

I feel the need to repeat; I consider the Healthcare Delivery System to be the Greatest Social (non-military, non-foreign policy) Responsibility for every Civilized Nation, because that System directly impacts the lives of every living person, plus those yet unborn. Yet, that System has been allowed to evolve into a poorly organized manner in every Civilized Nation. And spare me with the examples of some countries with very small populations, and nanny-styled forms of government. Every country on this planet with a large population is forced to admit that their current Healthcare System is rife with long-standing, inherent problems.

Healthcare experts have been talking about thousands of Needless Hospital Deaths for decades as if those numbers didn't represent real people whose lives were *needlessly cut short.*

Yet, the Healthcare Delivery System continues to be treated like an illegitimate child at a family reunion.

Open minds are what has been missing, and the basic failure to recognize that medicine is a scientific endeavor, and all science is made up of far more questions than answers. Open minds are necessary for effective discussion and dialogue, but I have found that open minds have been missing in the Quality of Care and Patient Safety army of experts, and Dr. Leape's 440-page book Making Healthcare Safe provides hard evidence of such absence. Each of those experts depicted in his book speaks with a level of conviction that fails to support the final judgement. Our current Healthcare Delivery System is sadly, no safer now than it was when those Harvard School of Public Health experts began their deep dive into upstate New York hospital patient records in the mid-1980s. Four decades later, and still patient beware.

Being the contrarian regarding critical issues is not fun, and I can only say that my intent is positive, and I believe there is an important distinction between being a positive contrarian to being a negative one. It is easy to become frustrated during a prolonged period of watching acclaimed experts continually ignore fundamental facts such as those that clearly support the understanding that each state is responsible to create and maintain an effective Healthcare Delivery System since each state long has been the source of authority of that system.

After my meeting in the CMS Headquarters in March 2020, and the absence of any interest or response to my meeting with the Chief of the Medical Staff and three of her Deputies my frustration led me to create a second edition of ***FIND THE BLACK BOX*** and include the following **2020 Preface.**

2020 Preface

FIND THE BLACK BOX, PREVENT NEEDLESS HOSPITAL DEATHS, and THE SOLUTION NO ONE ELSE IS TALKING ABOUT was first published in 2013, but my efforts to improve the current HEALTHCARE DELIVERY SYSTEM (HCDS) have continued, and my understanding of that enormous, and complex *system* has grown substantially. And the first issue that deserves close consideration is regarding the second sub-title.

THE SOLUTION NO ONE ELSE IS TALKING ABOUT: Not only has no one else been talking about the solution for how to make our current HCDS far better, none of the other Quality of Care and Patient Safety experts who have been publicly promising to create positive change in that *system* have shown the slightest interest in inviting me to join them in their quest for improvement, or even asked for more details about my offering.

Experts (those claiming expertise) not only should be challenged because no one person can know everything there is to know about enormous, complex issues, but every expert should seek to be challenged. Sadly, I have found the entire body of Quality of Care and Patient Safety army of experts to have bear-trap minds, and they are all snapped shut. My books and my offering are meant to be a courteous challenge to other experts, and my intent is to provide positive contributions to their ongoing efforts to make our current HCDS far better, and the next issue I submit for consideration is of the utmost importance.

The Healthcare Delivery System is the Greatest Social Responsibility of every Civilized Nation.

Every civilized nation's HCDS directly impacts every living person from first breath to last, plus those yet unborn. Yet I believe that every civilized nation's HCDS, particularly within those nations with sizable populations, will be found to be as unorganized, and ineffective where effectiveness is most important as our Nation's current HCDS, and factual evidence to support my contention is clearly evident for those who might seek to recognize such sad facts.

I have been attempting to courteously challenge, and seeking to engage high level political authorities, and healthcare experts since I wrote my 2nd book *MISDIAGNOSED! Why Current Health Care Change is Malpractice* in 2010, and I feel it will be enlightening to share some of my many efforts to help make Your and Your Loved One's HCDS far better.

My Bookends refer to personal efforts in 2010-11, and 2019-20 primarily because of the persons of highest authority I sought to engage with, and share my concerns, and expertise.

2010 Three Events:

"Even if we had a cure for cancer, we couldn't get it to the people because the current system is broken!" Dr. Spence Taylor, Chairman of the Committee seeking to establish a new medical school in Greenville SC in an interview with the Greenville Journal, April.

MISDIAGNOSED! WHY CURRENT HEALTH CARE CHANGE IS MALPRACTICE, my 2nd book was published in September. Nikki Haley was successfully elected Governor in November, and during her campaigns she said she would listen to anyone seeking to speak with her, and I believed her.

2011: Two Events

"There's no question that our nation's healthcare system is broken." Ingo Angermeier, President/CEO, Spartanburg Regional Hospital, and former President, South Carolina Hospital Association in a article he wrote published in the Greenville Magazine, April.

Governor Nikki Haley provided me with a 10-minute face-to-face meeting in August. I first showed her my back-to-back copies of Dr. Taylor's and Ingo's quotes, and a copy of my latest book, *MISDIAGNOSED!* I then told her that I could provide her with a detailed picture of her State's HCDS. She made no comment, and no offer to meet again.

2013. Governor Haley sent word she could not accept my offer, but no reason was given.

2020: Three Events

CMS Director Verma provided me with contact to her office at a brief face-to-face meeting in Greenville SC in December 2019.

This enabled me to meet with CMS Chief of Medical Staff Dr. Shari Ling, and other staff members at CMS Baltimore Headquarters for 1 hour on March 5, 2020.

I later established contact with CMS Innovation Center Director Brad Smith in May.

My email message to Director Verma, Dr. Ling, and Director Smith in June contained the following: I can provide a process for how to begin to create a 21st century Healthcare Delivery System (doctors, hospitals, and surgery centers). NO response to my offer has been received.

So, during a ten year span my offer to contribute to the efforts to make your and your loved one's HCDS far better have been rejected, first by then SC Governor Nikki Haley, and more recently by CMS Director Verma, and CMS Innovation Center Director Smith, all with NO reason given. But my contact with Nikki Haley had not ended.

STAND for AMERICA, c/o NIKKI HALEY, COLUMBIA, SC. (requesting donations), and I sent her instead the following letter:

> *Nikki Haley*
>
> *July 15, 2020*
>
> *Concerned Citizen,*
>
> *I doubt you remember our brief meeting in August 2011 therefore I have included some reminders of that meeting, and my thus far unsuccessful efforts to gain reasonable consideration from decision-makers at Federal, State, and Local levels for the past decade. I have found it exceedingly difficult to find people with open minds.*

I know why all the efforts to improve the quality of care and patient safety have been far more ineffective than promised, and also how to begin to create a 21st century HC Delivery System (doctors & hospitals) worthy of our Nation, but all of the experts appear to be too busy to show interest in my offerings.

Since our brief meeting in August 2011, I have published two new books.

Find The Black Box, Prevent Needless Hospital Deaths 2013 (web site .org)

Healthcare Warriors, Why and How to Become One 2019 (web site .org)

Three Events page is offered as the "bookends" of my efforts to courteously challenge decision-makers in Congress, SC Legislature, Federal Quality of Care Agencies, etc. during the period 2010-2020, and the response has been the same at every level of government: NO interest.

All the "experts" are forced to agree that the present HCDS is "broken", a very poor word for such a critical understanding, but the word most used. Yet none of those experts have the slightest interest in permitting me to contribute to their efforts to improve the current non-system.

I am writing this with the hope that you will personally have an opportunity to read it, because my plans are to begin to vigorously promote my books and my ideas regarding our current HCDS, why it is broken, and how to begin to correct that critical problem, and given an opportunity I will have this to say about you.

I have no personal animosity toward Governor/Ambassador Haley.

1. *I anticipate her 6-year term as SC Governor will be recorded in our State's History books in a very positive manner.*
2. *In my opinion, Governor Haley chose to be incompetent regarding her state's healthcare delivery system, and for*

more reasons than her failure to give even the slightest consideration to my 2011 offer to her regarding the SC HCDS.

I intend you NO disrespect, but our brief meeting was my first of many, many attempts to interact with decision-makers at every level of government, and with the same failed result during the past several years.

The Healthcare Delivery System (IMO) is the greatest social responsibility of every civilized nation because that "System" directly impacts every living person, from first breath to last, plus those yet unborn. I can provide a historical timeline, from the first day, of the evolution of our current HCDS, and it is NOT a pretty picture. Our greatest social responsibility has been allowed to evolve with NO master plan, and is now unorganized, and highly dysfunctional, and the reasons why are clearly evident to those who choose to look.

It is evident that you seek to remain a major player on the National scene, and therefore you not only should be challenged, but you should seek to be challenged. And I am taking this opportunity to courteously challenge you regarding our Nation's and our State's HCDS.

I can tell you things about you and your loved one's HCDS that no one else will tell you. But first you must have a desire to gain knowledge of those truths.

My Second Offer: IF you, and others wish to understand why our current HCDS is and has always been far less than it could or should be, and how to begin to create a far better system, I am available, but not optimistic.

It must be remembered that there is nothing more difficult to plan, more doubtful of success, no more dangerous to manage than a new system. For the initiator has the enmity of all who would profit by the preservation of the old institution, and merely lukewarm defenders in those who gain by the new one. Machiavelli

Sadly, his prophetic assessment of human nature is as true today as it was in Florence Italy over 500 years ago,

> *and decision makers still don't get it. No one knows everything about enormous, complex "systems", and that is why it requires a collaboration of efforts to begin to make positive change. I am simply trying to contribute to the efforts to make our Nation's and our State's HCDS far better, and I know how to do that.*
>
> *Sincerely,*
> **Ira E. Williams**

Either her staff in Columbia trashed my letter, or she again felt I deserved NO response.

While my decade-long Bookends demonstrate my attempts to engage persons at the highest state, and highest federal levels of government, and those persons total disinterest, they only represent a very small number of attempts I have made, and continue to make seeking an opportunity to contribute to the efforts to make our current HCDS far better, and since FTBB was first published in 2013 I will limit further examples of my attempts to the past seven years.

2014 I was a Keynote presenter at the 3-day 11th World Healthcare Congress, DC in April, and was probably the only one to speak about each state's responsibility for the HCDS. I also joined the Society to Improve Diagnosis in Medicine (SIDM) and in Sept. attended the 3-day Annual Meeting in Atlanta where I gave a Board member a 2-page paper prior to their morning Board meeting. No Board member spoke to me after they came out of their Board meeting, and I accepted their rejection, and returned home mid-day of the second day.

2016 In July I traveled to DC and attended all day meetings, first at the National Academy of Medicine (NAM), and 2 days later at AHRQ in Rockville MD where I presented both Agencies' Presidents with a 1-page letter offering to provide details regarding my opinion of the 2 Greatest Healthcare Mistakes in the HCDS. My request for consideration was not rejected, but simply ignored by both Federal Agencies' Senior Staff.

2017. I returned to DC for a one-day SIDM meeting at the NAM where I challenged all attendees at the first morning Q&A, and again at the mid-afternoon Q&A. NAM retains videos of their all-day meetings, and my participation should be available if requested.

2018. I challenged my friend and State Representative for his seat in the SC Legislature, not with the thought of winning, but only seeking to participate in an open debate that would allow me to openly discuss the current status of our State's HCDS. But the City Leaders in both Mauldin and Simpsonville (suburbs of Greenville) made sure that there would be no public debate by the candidates. The result was I had wasted a lot of money and good will to no avail. I also released my 4th book *HEALTHCARE WARRIORS, WHY AND HOW TO BECOME ONE* in eBook form only at that time, followed by print in 2019, and audio in 2020.

Governor McMaster, who had succeeded Governor Haley when she became UN Ambassador in 2016 was seeking to remain SC Governor, and he had chosen Pamela Evette, a very successful businesswoman to be his Lt. Governor. Mrs. Evette kindly allowed me to meet with her and her Administrative Assistant at her business office near Greenville SC in August, before the election. The three of us spent 1 hour in a small room where I presented copies of my 4 books, Dr. Makary's book *UNACCOUNTABLE*, and many documents including the two quotes by Dr. Spence Taylor, and Ingo Angermeier from 2010, and 2011 each stating that the "system is broken", and my offer to then Governor Haley that I could provide a detail picture of the SC HCDS.

The three things that I have taken from that lengthy exchange are Mrs. (now SC Lt. Governor) Evette said that Dr. Taylor was a friend, I left copies of all of the books, and all of the additional supporting literature, and SC Lt. Governor Evette, and re-elected SC Governor McMaster have never requested that I provide them with additional information.

Dr. Spence Taylor would later become President/CEO of Greenville Health System, the largest such system in the state until his retirement in late 2019, and there is no evidence that

Dr. Taylor ever felt he had a responsibility to tell the citizens of South Carolina; How is their HCDS "broken", Why is their HCDS 'broken", and What, if anything, had he and others been doing to "fix" their HCDS? Recognition that our Nation's, and every State's HCDS is, and has always been "broken" for the past several decades is well established. But none of the Quality of Care and Patient Safety experts, including the Federal Quality of Care Agencies, seem to want to talk about how to begin to create a far better system than I have been offering for the past decade.

During the past decade I have made many attempts to share my concerns with state legislators, particularly in the Greenville/Spartanburg SC area, and I was always met with complete disinterest. The SC Legislature has 27 standing committees, 14 in the Senate, and 13 in the House of Representatives, and the word HEALTHCARE does not appear on the page. Readers should assume that the SC Legislature is merely a snapshot of other state legislatures and begin to ask questions where they live. Machiavelli was right, contrarians can expect to receive great opposition, and scant support, as is clearly evident throughout history.

My 2020 BOOKEND

Center for Medicare and Medicaid Services dominates what is allowed, and what is not allowed in most hospitals in the Nation, and their Headquarters outside Baltimore MD is like a giant ant hill with "worker ants" making policy, and shuffling papers from one part of the building to another, but it appears that IF a new idea is not one of their ideas it is not worthy of consideration. CMS Verma became a part of President Trump's Administration because she had been Vice President Pence's Indiana Department of Health Director, and therefore she has great experience regarding the HCDS at the state level, and one should assume that her HCDS had critical shortcomings at that level of patient care. Yet CMS Verma, and her Innovation Center Director Smith have NO interest in what I might have to offer to the efforts to make our current HCDS far better. But I did not end my efforts to courteously challenge "experts" while waiting to see if the CMS decision-makers might open their minds.

MISTREATED, WHY WE THINK WE'RE GETTING GOOD HEALTH CARE—AND WHY WE'RE USUALLY WRONG, Dr. Robert Pearl, M.D. 2017.

This 2020 Preface is being written in November, and I had just belatedly discovered, and read two books, both written in 2017 while writing this Preface.

Dr. Robert Pearl is the former CEO of The Permanente Medical Group (1999-2017), the nation's largest medical group, and former president of The Mid-Atlantic Permanente Medical Group (2009-2017). In these roles he led 10,000 physicians, 38,000 staff and was responsible for the nationally recognized medical care of five million Kaiser Permanente members on the west and east coasts.

Named one of *Modern Healthcare's* 50 most influential physician leaders, Pearl is an advocate for the power of integrated, prepaid, technologically advanced, and physician-led healthcare delivery. He serves as a clinical professor of plastic surgery at Stanford University School of Medicine and is on the faculty of the Stanford Graduate School of Business, where he teaches courses on strategy and leadership, and lectures on information technology and health care policy. (his web site).

I sent a message to Dr. Pearl on his web site that included the following: I found your book to be an indictment of all of the efforts to improve the quality of care and patient safety during the past several decades, and all of the "experts" who have contributed to those efforts, AND I believe your indictment was proper, and correct. I was surprised and pleased that he responded.

*Hello **Dr. Williams**,*

I'm sorry that what I wrote came across as "an indictment of all the efforts to improve the quality of care and patient safety during the past decades." There are many ways in which we have improved. Having said that, the fact our nation only controls hypertension 55% of the time and screens for colon cancer less than 70% of the time concerns me. And medical errors and avoidable complications from chronic diseases are in the hundreds of thousands. The four pillars I offer have been effective at lowering deaths from heart attacks, sepsis, strokes, and cancer by over 30% in various medical groups and organizations.

At the same time, I always want to learn more, so if you have better solutions than the ones I propose, please send them to me and I will read the material in depth.

Thanks,
Robbie

Robbie,

Thank you for responding. My intentions are positive. I have written four books on the HCDS. All self-published due to a lack of obtaining literary agent support. The consensus is The System is Broken, but there is little detailed discussion about How is it Broken, why is it Broken, and more importantly, How can we begin to create a far more worthy "System". I can answer all parts of that assessment.

This thing we all have become compelled to call a "system" has always been devoid of any true systematic characteristics, and I can speak to that in detail, but not in brief soundbites.

Second Great Mistake: States, each state, are responsible to create and maintain an effective HCDS, and no governor or state legislator has ever sought to fulfill that critical responsibility. All medical care is local and states license doctors and hospitals, and surgery centers (we oral surgeons established the credibility of surgery centers long before you "real doctors" recognized their value). Yet during the past ten years I appear to be the only one speaking about the state of responsibility.

I was in the CMS Hedqs. outside Baltimore March 5th this year, and I have informed CMS Director Verma, and CMS Innovation Center Director Smith that I can provide a process for how to begin to create a 21st century HCDS, but I have received NO response. I was probably the only speaker at the 11th World HC Congress in

DC in 2014 who spoke about each state's responsibility, and I attempted to speak to you, but was unable.

I am just a DDS like your late father (board certified oral & maxillofacial surgeon and anesthesiologist) and I truly believe I have a better understanding of the current HCDS, AND how to begin to create a far better system than anyone else, and every time I say that I mean it as a courteous challenge. NAM has video evidence of me challenging a room full of experts twice at the SIDM meeting on July 17, 2017. Beth McGlynn was there, and she accepted a copy of my 3rd book Find The Black Box several years ago. Ask her.

I am attaching My Offer and hope you will accept. Robbie, I don't mean to offend, and I am not a bomb-thrower. I just want to participate in the efforts to make our HCDS far better, but no one seems to want to accept me.

Ira

Ira,

Like you, I don't believe we have a system. In fact, in Mistreated, I label it a 19th century cottage industry. Like you I recognize the issues with trying to provide healthcare to 300 million people and delegating it to 50 different entities (states). [He sees but doesn't recognize the problem.]

I read a huge amount of material from people with interesting and important ideas—and learn from all. As I said, I'd be happy to read whatever you choose to send me. My opinions often reflect multiple inputs. I try to credit people in my writing but find that many ideas overlap.

Robbie

Robbie

Your first few words in your message astound me. Recognition of that FACT by everyone claiming to contribute to the efforts to improve the current non-system must be the first step, but that recognition has only been given passive lip-service since To Err Is

Human stated such a possibility on the first page of the Introduction. Dr. Leape told the Senate HELP Subcommittee the plan to adopt safety measures from commercial aviation, and the chemical, and nuclear power industries in Jan. 2000 immediately after publication of To Err Is Human, and twenty years later we are still where we were back then regarding improved quality of care and patient safety at the doctor/patient interface, as you describe in your book.

As a top HC leader in California, can you describe in detail your state's HCDS; identity each component that contributes to that "system", provide some detail regarding each component's contribution, and the Kicker, identify any systematic collaboration between various components necessary to be classified as a true system? We all continue to lie to ourselves, and any potential audience every time we use the word system in relation to HC and wonder why no real progress is being made in the efforts to make the current system (there I go again) better.

And I was disappointed you made no mention of my attachment. Have you had similar offers from others? The next time you reference your desire to help make things better in memory of your father I hope you will re-read my offer list.

Ira

Robbi,

I meant to add—I love this and hope you will continue with the exchange.

Ira

Ira

In the book, I point out many of the areas of quality failure and reference "To Err is Human." I appreciate your offer to provide your thoughts (and data) on the topics. I felt I was responding by leaving it to you to decide what you chose to send me.

I receive dozens of similar offers from smart, insightful doctors and policy experts each week, and wouldn't sleep if I pursued all of the offers similar to yours. I've probably read 50 books written by others and mailed to me since Mistreated. My solution is to leave it to those who write to decide what they feel would be most interesting and helpful.

I think my dad would be pleased with the breadth of feedback I've read, and how I've used it to advance my thinking and writing since the book's publication. Most of those who have sent me material wish I would dive deeper into their recommendations. My approach is what has been labelled "wisdom of the crowd." To that end, I've tried to combine the different ideas with my own. In the end, we don't make much progress in the healthcare system because people (insurers, hospital administrators, specialists, etc.) are not very interested in doing so. As in so many areas, there are multiple solutions that could lead to improvement, but all will fail if people don't choose to pursue them. Like you, at this point in my career (no longer being a CEO) I can encourage and point the way, but I can't force leaders to go forward.

Robbie

Robbie

So, I guess you are content with leaving the Public with your book's Sub-Title; Why we think we're getting good healthcare and why we're usually wrong. Tell Beth McGlynn I said hello.

Ira

I hope readers noticed that in his second message to me he stated, "Like you, I don't believe we have a system. In fact, in Mistreated, I label it a 19th century cottage industry." How can experts acknowledge that the current system is a non-system, and continuously ignore the importance of that critical understanding? Use of the word "system" regarding healthcare is a LIE!

EXPERTS with bear-trap minds, and they are ALL CLOSED!

CMS Dir. Verma, CMS Innovation Center Dir. Smith, Dr. Robert Pearl, SC Governor, and former Ambassador Haley, and current SC Governor McMaster, and Lt. Governor Evette show

NO interest in the well-documented evidence that you and your loved one's HCDS is and has always been broken. I have been offering a process for how to begin to create a far better system for the past ten years, and those named above, and many others have shown NO interest.

The second book:

MALPRACTICE, A Neurosurgeon Reveals

How Our Health-Care System Puts Patients at Risk, LAWRENCE SCHLACHTER, M.D. 2017

I met Dr. Schlachter, and two other people for lunch, and discussions regarding my book *FIND THE BLACK BOX* in September 2015, and he stated he was writing a book on medical malpractice at that time. His book, and his experiences as both a surgeon and a plaintiff's attorney in malpractice cases have given him great knowledge and understanding regarding the fundamental unfairness that has been inherent in medical malpractice litigation for centuries in our Nation. But his knowledge and understanding about the current system has not provided him with an understanding of how to replace that system with an effective medical peer review system whereby doctors can fairly judge other doctors regarding questionable patient care. I can provide such a system of fair medica peer review and said so in my first book *FIRST DO NO HARM, THE CURE FOR MEDICAL MALPRACTICE,* 2004.

I have judged other doctors (MD & DDS) in civil court proceedings regarding questionable patient care, and by doing so, I have come to know how practitioners can fairly judge other doctors. The problem is that is the last thing doctors would desire to have. Simply stated, doctors are never trained on how to judge other doctor's questionable care because throughout the history of the medical profession doctors' basic inclinations have been to shelter such doctors and rely on a highly flawed medical malpractice litigation system that allows them to protect their fellow members. In every case in Madison WI that I testified as the second surgeon in malpractice civil court proceeding against MD surgeons involving gross malpractice in each case, the hospital medical staffs, and other doctors, including University of Wisconsin Department heads did everything they could to protect the offending surgeons up to, and including lying under oath. The Medical Profession, including every association, state medical society, and state medical examining board have supported a litigation system that if examined closely might be considered a criminal enterprise. Yet that system has been tolerated by every level of government for centuries.

Another, and possibly the most important book in this Preface: UNDERSTANDING PATIENT SAFETY, Robert M. Wachter, MD, Kiran Gupta, MD, MPH, 3rd Edition, 2018.

This is a large paperback book containing 3 Sections, and 22 Chapters in its 510 pages.

Section III: SOLUTIONS contains 10 of those 22 Chapters, and the author's inclusion in the book's PREFACE as to the need for this 3rd Edition is noteworthy.

The first edition of *Understanding Patient Safety* was published in 2007, and the second in 2012. In preparing this third edition five years later, we were impressed by the maturation of the safety field. Between the first and second edition, for example, there were fundamental changes in our understanding of safety targets, with a shift to a focus on harm rather than errors. We saw the emergence of checklists as a key tool in safety. New safety-oriented practices, such as rapid response teams and medication reconciliation, became commonplace. The digitization of medical practice was just beginning to gain steam, but most doctor's offices and hospitals remained paper bound. Between 2012 and today, the most impressive change has been the wide-spread computerization of the healthcare system.

[**Note:** *There is NO mention of each state's responsibility, and also the consistent use of the word "system" throughout their book while there have been some suggestions that the current "system" is actually a "non-system", a critical realization IF proven to be true, and it is true.*]

Dr. Wachter and my brief face-to-face meeting here in Greenville SC in 2010 is described in some detail in this book's

1st Edition INTRODUCTION, and during our brief conversation he admitted he had a problem trying to make his, and other's "solutions" become reality, and I told him, "I can solve that problem". We followed our conversation with a short exchange of email messages, but NO invitation for me to join him in his efforts to make the current system better. Maybe some of my solutions could be included in their next edition.

In 2013 Dr. Wachter gave me permission to use some of his journal articles, and a few of his **AHRQ Web M&M, morbidity and mortality** interviews he periodically conducted with selected patient safety experts during the past decade. Interestingly, at least to me, after I had told him "I can solve that problem" in 2010 he never felt the need to request to interview me. But I hope readers will take particular interest in those few M&M interviews I included.

Semmelweis, Pasteur, Lister, are just a few of the names of those who made great contributions in the on-going efforts to make the delivery of patient care safer, and more effective, and each of those renowned individual's personal histories demonstrate the consistent pattern of obstruction, and denigration evident throughout the history of the medical profession. Contrarian beliefs, even when supported by strong evidence, have consistently been resisted, and opposed, and such unprofessional behavior has continued to be evident during the past decade. But I keep knocking on the door.

I have been saying for the past ten years in my books, personal challenges to Patient Safety experts, and political leaders at every level regarding my belief that there has been NO real, and effective improvement in the efforts to begin to improve the quality of care and patient safety during the past several decades due to the failure by all such experts to recognize or ignore.

The Two Greatest Mistakes regarding the Healthcare Delivery System:
Each state is responsible for creating and maintaining an effective Healthcare Delivery System.

The current HCDS is, and has always been, devoid of any *systematic characteristics,* and effective accountability will always be impossible to impose without the creation of a clearly defined organizational structure, with effective points of delegated authority necessary for effective accountability to exist.

Dr. Marty Makary's two books, *UNACCOUNTABLE* 2012, and *WHAT PRICE WE PAY* 2019, and Drs. Wachter and Gupta's *UNDERSTANDING PATIENT SAFETEY* 2018, are excellent examples of all of those authors and their books who have been capable of identifying the many problems within the current "system", but have been incapable of identifying the root causes of why NO real improvement in the quality of care and patient safety has been made, and NO suggestion for how to begin to create a 21st century Healthcare Delivery System worthy of our Nation. In fact, they never seem to talk about creating a 21st century HCDS.

Drs. Wachter and Grupta's final statement in their book's CONCLUSION speaks volumes.

"We still have much to do before we get there." They recognized "something is still missing" in their on-going efforts to improve the quality of care and patient safety, BUT they still are unable to identify those missing key elements. Perhaps IF Dr. Wachter had taken far more interest in what I might have to offer to their efforts following our verbal exchange here in Greenville SC ten years ago, and invited me to participate in their efforts, we, they, might be further along in their quest for greater understanding.

I am the only quality of care and patient safety expert who has been saying that I can provide clear evidence of what has always been missing in the decades-old efforts to make our current HCDS better, and I am also the only expert who has been saying that I know how to begin to create a 21st century HCDS, but NO ONE seemed interested.

I want to close this 2020 Preface with two final pages in which I seek to identify multiple, specific challenges to members of that vast army of Quality of Care and Patient Safety experts who have been promising quality of care improvements for over three decades and have little to show for those efforts.

I KNOW WHY OUR CURRENT HCDS HAS ALWAYS FAILED THE PUBLIC, AND I KNOW HOW TO BEGIN TO CREATE A FAR BETTER "SYSTEM". MY PROBEM HAS BEEN MY INABILITY TO FIND EXPERTS WITH OPEN MINDS WHO ARE RECEPTIVE TO BEING CHALLENGED IN A COURTEOUS AND POSITIVE MANNER.

Questions Quality of Care Experts never asked, therefore never answered.
1. **Is the current HCDS the Greatest Social Responsibility?**
2. **How is the current HCDS broken?**
3. **Why is the current HCDS broken?**
4. **How should a process to improve the current HCDS begin?**

Answers
1. The next time a reader or loved one becomes a patient in a hospital they should ask themselves what social responsibility so directly impacts every living person? None.
2. Despite having the greatest HCDS on the Planet, when individual patient care falls below an acceptable standard of care there is rarely effective accountability. American Medical Association (AMA) has always left the Public with Sue of Forget It, and the AMA definition of medical malpractice is "treatment beneath a standard of care *set by the law*." The failure to provide effective accountability involving instances of questionable patient care is how the current HCDS has always failed the people it was created to serve.
3. Two Greatest Healthcare Mistakes:
    a. Failure to recognize that since states license doctors and hospitals, each state is responsible to create and maintain an effective HCDS.
    b. Failure to recognize that the current "system" is devoid of any systematic characteristics and has

always lacked a clearly defined organization structure necessary for effective accountability.
4. First there must be recognition of each state's responsibility, and then seek to describe any state's current HCDS by identifying each component that contributes to that system and seek to identify any evidence of multiple component collaboration that might provide evidence of a true "system". There should be NO attempt to begin to create a new "system" without first creating a well-defined picture of each state's current "system".

"Education is primarily a State and local responsibility in the United States." The Federal Role in Education, U. S. Department of Education, April 2019.

The same recognition is critically needed regarding our current HCDS.

I have been attempting to contribute to the efforts to improve the HCDS at both Federal and State levels, and I have been constantly and consistently denied such an opportunity. My self-published books have been my primary tools to try to make my views known. But there are other subjects closely related to the efforts to improve the current HCDS that I have not yet written about.

Books started, but unwritten:
The Three Men Who Opened the Door to Modern Medicine

The Historical Timeline of the Evolution of Our Current HCDS.

I can provide the following expertise.
Regarding How to Begin to Create a 21st Century HCDS

1. Define and describe the 2 Greatest Healthcare Mistakes regarding the current Healthcare Delivery System. (Updated to 3 Greatest Mistakes)
2. Describe why the multiple Federal Quality of Care and Patient Safety agencies created by Congress have been so ineffective for the past several decades.

3. A detailed picture of any state's current Healthcare Delivery System (doctors & hospitals), including further steps toward creating a new HCDS.
4. A historical timeline of the evolution of our Nation's current Healthcare Delivery System from its first day, and it is NOT a pretty picture.

Regarding How to Provide Effective Medical Staff Accountability

1. A peer review system for how doctors can <u>fairly</u> judge the patient care capability of other doctors, but that is the last thing doctors would wish to have.
2. I can demonstrate unethical and unprofessional conduct within the medical staff, and by others, in every hospital in the Nation.
3. I can identify the critical medical practitioner responsibility that has been missing or consistently ignored in every hospital medical staff.
4. The imperative responsibilities of every practitioner in every surgery center.
5. How the AMA definition of medical malpractice demonstrates that profession's abandonment of the Public.
6. Clear evidence, in their own words, how the American Hospital Association and their 50 state components have been an enemy of the Public.

Other HC experts have been talking about the Problem(s)—I can and want to talk about the Solution—but funny thing—I haven't been able to find any other "expert" who wishes to participate in such a dialogue.

I am the author of 4 books on the Healthcare Delivery System, and I challenge other Healthcare experts regarding the above assertions.

Frustration personified.

This is being written during the beginning of the much-too-long race for the White House, and the early stages of the multitude of candidates seeking the presidential nomination. I have been attending several of the early visits by various candidates in my area of South Carolina, and one thing has stood out to me during all those campaign events so far; the subject of healthcare is never mentioned. No one in South Carolina will touch on that subject, and so far, none of the candidates have either.

The Healthcare System directly impacts the lives of every living person, plus those yet unborn, and the multitude of problems within that System are clearly evident. Yet, that subject seems to be a proverbial "political third rail", and with the caution that anyone seeking political office who touches that subject will die politically.

www.ingramcontent.com/pod-product-compliance
Lightning Source LLC
LaVergne TN
LVHW011938070526
838202LV00054B/4709